Hystories

Hysterical Epidemics and Modern Media

Elaine Showalter

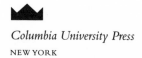

Columbia University Press

NEW YORK

Columbia University Press
Publishers Since 1893
New York   Chichester, West Sussex

Library of Congress Cataloging-in-Publication Data
Showalter, Elaine.
    Hystories : hysterical epidemics and modern media / Elaine
    Showalter.
        p.   cm.
    Includes bibliographical references and index.
    ISBN 0-231-10458-8 (alk. paper) — ISBN 0-231-10459-6 (pbk.)
    1. Hysteria, Epidemic.   2. Hysteria (Social psychology).
    3. Popular culture.   I. Title.
RC532.S46   1997
616.85'24—dc20   96-44108
                                                                        CIP

♾

Casebound editions of Columbia University Press books are printed on
permanent and durable acid-free paper.
Printed in the United States of America
c 10 9 8 7 6 5 4 3 2 1
p 10 9 8 7 6 5 4 3 2 1

For English, Vinca, and Michael

Contents

Preface to the Paperback Edition

When I finished writing *Hystories* in fall 1996, I noted that although some hysterical epidemics seemed to be waning, others were springing up to take their places. A year later, I am nonetheless surprised at the hystories that have emerged since the book's publication. Who would have guessed that members of the Heaven's Gate cult would commit mass suicide in hope of joining an alien spaceship they believed lay behind the tail of the Halle-Bopp comet? That the fiftieth anniversary of Roswell would become a media circus, and that the town would turn into an alien theme park? That a Wisconsin doctor would be sued for diagnosing a patient with 120 personalities, including a duck, and for billing her insurance company for group therapy? That rumors about the fate of TWA Flight 800 would still be circulating on the Internet? That a doctor in Los Angeles would claim he caught Gulf War Syndrome from his patients and it made his teeth fall out, and an ex-army nurse who never went to the Gulf would be sure she had given GWS to her dog? Or, uncannily and tragically, that Princess Diana, who had courageously overcome her own hysterical eating disorder, would die at the Salpetriere Hospital in Paris, where modern hysteria began; that journalists would be asking about the hysterical reaction to her death; and that conspiracy theories about it would be raging?

I anticipated that *Hystories* would upset some special-interest groups, and it did. Angry responses come with the territory of this applied research, and have to be expected by anyone who challenges the belief systems of sufferers. Dr. Paul McHugh, Director of the Department of Psychiatry and Behavioral Science at the Johns Hopkins School of Medicine, has written that challenges to such systems are "not for the faint-hearted or inexperienced. They seldom quickly succeed because they are often misrepresented as ignorant or, in the cant word of our day, uncaring." In a 1997 study of online support groups used by chronic fatigue syndrome patients, Kathyryn P. Davison and James W. Pennebaker reported that on the Internet, "discussions of chronic fatigue authors who include in their writing suspected psychological factors or psychosocial treatment strategies are viewed as anathema, practically subhuman in their callous and ignorant statements."

But I didn't predict that I would become the subject of conspiracy theories myself, that I would be accused of writing the book with secret "major corporate funding" and attacked as a "fascist" trying to "bolster a flagging career in academia." I didn't foresee that my editors at Columbia University Press would be called "cunt-sucking maggots to let this one slither through." I didn't anticipate that people would bombard me with hate mail, offer me blood transfusions, advise me to get a bodyguard, threaten to rip me apart, or warn me of assassination unless I recanted. In fact, although another year's accumulated scientific evidence has supported my arguments, the inflammatory reaction to the book from some quarters has only confirmed my analysis of hysterical epidemics of denial, projection, accusation, and blame.

On the other hand, I've had the opportunity to meet and correspond with many doctors, scientists, journalists, scholars, and government officials who have extended and enriched my understanding of these syndromes. These personal exchanges with other investigators have strengthened my resolve to make connections between my academic research and controversial public issues of our time. The expansion of the Internet and the World Wide Web have made medical research and information more accessible than ever before, and e-mail has made it possible for me to be in dialogue with colleagues all over the world.

With regard to chronic fatigue syndrome, little has changed. Much-touted medical studies suggesting that neurally mediated hypotension, or brain lesions, or an enzyme, could be definitively connected to the syndrome have not been replicated or proven, and the community remains resistant to psychological treatments and interpretations. Meanwhile, patients tell stories of prolonged illness, worsening disability, and deepening distress. The CFS diagnosis is increasingly being applied to adolescents.

As for Gulf War Syndrome, the real gulf is still the one between alleged causes and proven effects. Despite the conclusions of five U.S. independent commissions that there is no single illness and that stress is the major factor, conspiracy theories about Gulf War Syndrome continue to flourish. Suspicions were undoubtedly reinforced on July 24, 1997, when CIA and Department of Defense officials announced that the vaporized sarin plume from the explosion at Kamisayah may have reached 99,000 service members. But whether 100 or 100,000 troops may have been exposed to vaporized sarin, the likelihood that it could have caused any long-term symptoms remains remote. Nerve gases cause symptoms immediately upon exposure, and there was not a single complaint of nerve gas poisoning during the conflict, though such poisoning causes unmissable symptoms: pinpoint pupils, runny nose, eye pain, sweating, nausea, diarrhea, convulsions, and wheezing. In addition, three decades of research on nerve gases have produced no evidence of long-term damage from low-level exposure. In the U.K., where troops were not exposed to any nerve gas, Gulf War Syndrome has been blamed on everything from flea collars to sheep dip; but although British and American conspiracy theories of government cover-ups continue to diverge in their hypotheses, the overall belief in government cover-up remains unshakable.

With regard to recovered memories, ritual abuse charges, and multiple personalities, however, the tide seems to have turned. Courts are continuing to reverse decisions, and in an few highly publicized cases, day-care center workers convicted of abusing children, such as the "Edenton Seven" in North Carolina, have been released from prison and charges against them have been dropped. Yet many of these people's lives have been wrecked by false allegations. In the U.K., local health-care officials have still not released a highly critical report about a satanic ritual abuse scare of 1989. Television documentaries, tabloid newspapers, and sensational movies continue to spread the imagery of recovered memory, Satanism, and alien abduction around the world. If, as some polls claim, millions of Americans still believe in alien abduction, we have a long way still to go before credulity, superstition, and hysterical epidemics are on the wane. Confronting these syndromes may indeed generate heat, but without heat, there can be no light.

Elaine Showalter
October 1997

Acknowledgments

Ⅰt was a happy day in 1978 when I first began working at the Wellcome Institute for the History of Medicine in London—an ace caff, a great staff, and a rather nice library attached. Sally Bragg has always made me feel welcome at the Wellcome and helped me make the most of its amazing resources. I'm grateful for the generosity and example of the Wellies, especially Bill Bynum, Roy Porter, Michael J. Clark, and Julia Sheppard. Many friends and colleagues in England aided and encouraged my work, even when they disagreed with my conclusions; my thanks to Juliet Mitchell, Susie Orbach, Lisa Tickner, John Forrester, Lisa Appignanesi, Louise Armstrong, Lisa Jardine, John Clay, Sally Alexander, Linda Grant, Ann Dally, Sarah Dunant, Diane Middlebrook, Anna Furse, Jacqueline Rose, Barbara Taylor, Marina Warner, and Michael Robinson. Erica Davies and Ivan Ward at the Freud Museum organized important symposia on hysteria today. In Paris, Sherrill Mulhern shared her remarkable collection of tapes and books; Jan Goldstein and Rae Beth Gordon offered valuable scholarly advice, and Catherine Saint Louis helped me track down treasures at the Bibliothèque Nationale.

At Princeton University, the Council for Research in the Humanities and Social Sciences has funded my research travel over the past several years. New Hysterian friends, especially Martha Noel Evans, Sander Gilman, Mark Micale, George Rousseau, Dianne Hunter, and Ian Hacking, have been ideal members of a vital, although far-flung, community of scholars. Stuart Burrows found stacks of references at the British Library and on the Internet. I have been blessed with a wonderful family, to whom I have dedicated this book, and with friends never too busy to listen, talk, or e-mail: Michael Cadden, Wendy Martin, Joyce Carol Oates, Larry Danson, Richard Kaye, and Carol Smith. My literary agents, Elaine Markson and Mary Clemmey, deserve thanks for years of good advice and advocacy. Finally, my brilliant and meticulous editor, M. Mark, made me account for every sentence, and Jennifer Crewe and Anne McCoy at Columbia University Press and Tanya Stobbs at Picador saw this project through its many stages with exemplary patience, professionalism, and panache.

Hystories

PART ONE

Histories

I

The Hysterical Hot Zone

In the Midwest, a nurse with chronic fatigue syndrome commits suicide with the help of Dr. Jack Kevorkian. In Yorkshire, a young Gulf War veteran struggles with a mysterious illness that has destroyed his marriage and his career. In California, an executive is disgraced after his daughter, who has been treated by her therapist with the hypnotic drug sodium amytal, says he abused her when she was a child; the court later awards him half a million dollars' damages. In Massachusetts, a Pulitzer Prize–winning Harvard professor claims that little gray aliens are visiting the United States and performing sexual experiments on thousands of Americans. In Oklahoma, accused bomber Timothy McVeigh tells his lawyers that the government planted a surveillance microchip in his buttocks during the Gulf War. In Montana, right-wing militias announce that the federal government, armed with bombs and black helicopters, is chemically altering the blood of U.S. citizens as part of its conspiracy to create a New World Order.

These sensational cases exemplify individual hysterias connecting with modern social movements to produce psychological epidemics. In books like Laurie Garrett's *The Coming Plague* (1994) and Richard Preston's *The Hot Zone* (1994), we've learned a lot about large-scale viral epidemics caused by killer microbes from the rain forest and the jungle. Fifty years ago scientists believed that antibiotics had conquered infectious disease and that the age of epidemics had passed into history. According to Garrett, these "boosters of the 1950s and early 1960s had some basis, born of ignorance, for their optimism; they knew comparatively little about genetics, microbial evolution, the human immune system, or disease ecology."[1] But infectious diseases had not been vanquished; they have proved remarkably resistant to medical triumphs and medical complacency. From Toxic Shock Syndrome to AIDS and the Ebola virus, emergent and resurgent diseases threaten societies that have believed themselves immune from pandemics.

Just as scientists prematurely proclaimed infectious diseases to be dead, so too psychiatrists prematurely announced the death of hysteria. In her 1965 study, Ilza Veith marveled at the "nearly total disappearance" of the disorder.[2] "Where has all the hysteria gone?" psychologist Roberta Satow asked a decade later.[3] Some doctors explained that the diagnostic tools of modern medicine had conquered hysteria by identifying it as unrecognized organic illness. A number of historians and sociologists argued that hysteria was really a Victorian disorder, a female reaction to sexual repression and limited opportunities, which diminished with the advent of modern feminism. Many psychiatrists believed that widespread awareness of Freudian psychoanalysis had made somatic conversion hysterias like limps and paralyses unfeasible as expressions of anxiety. According to the British analyst Harold Mersky in *The Analysis of Hysteria* (1978), conversion hysterias occur only in psychoanalytically unsophisticated areas such as East Africa, South Korea, Sri Lanka, or Nigeria. Whatever the cause, "hysteria is dead, that is certain," wrote the French medical historian Étienne Trillat, "and it has taken its secrets with it to the grave."[4]

But hysteria has not died. It has simply been relabeled for a new era. While Ebola virus and Lassa fever remain potential, psychological plagues at the end of the twentieth century are all too real. In the 1990s, the United States has become the hot zone of psychogenic diseases, new and mutating forms of hysteria amplified by modern communications and fin de siècle anxiety. Contemporary hysterical patients blame external sources—a virus, sexual molestation, chemical warfare, satanic conspiracy, alien infiltration—for psychic problems. A century after Freud, many people still reject psychological explanations for symptoms; they believe psychosomatic disorders are illegitimate and search for physical evidence that firmly places cause and cure outside the self.

When well-meaning crusaders see hysterical syndromes in the context of social crises and then publicize their views through modern communications networks, these misconceptions can give rise to epidemics and witch-hunts. In *The Pursuit of the Millennium*, the historian Norman Cohn describes the paranoias that accompany apocalyptic moments. "Those who are first attracted," he writes, "will mostly be people who seek a sanction for the emotional needs generated by their own unconscious conflicts. It is as though units of paranoia hitherto diffused through the population suddenly coalesce to form a new entity: a collective paranoiac fanaticism. But these first followers, precisely because they are true believers, can endow their new movement with such confidence, energy and ruthlessness that it will attract into its wake vast multitudes of people who are themselves not at all paranoid but simply harassed, hungry or frightened." When "a paranoiac mass movement captures political power," Cohn warns, disaster follows.[5]

Cohn writes about the year 1000 but he could be describing the mood right now. In the interaction between 1990s millennial panic, new psychotherapies, religious fundamentalism, and American political paranoia, we can see the crucible of virulent hysterias in our own time. The heroes and heroines of 1990s hysteria call themselves traumatists and ufologists, experiencers and abductees, survivors and survivalists. As their syndromes evolve, they grow from microtales of individual affliction to panics fueled by rumors about medical, familial, community, or governmental conspiracy. As the panic reaches epidemic proportions, hysteria seeks out scapegoats and enemies—from unsympathetic doctors, abusive fathers, and working mothers to devil-worshiping sadists, curious extraterrestrials, and evil governments.

Hystories

Hysteria not only survives in the 1990s, it is more contagious than in the past. Infectious diseases spread by ecological change, modern technology, urbanization, jet travel, and human interaction. Infectious epidemics of hysteria spread by stories circulated through self-help books, articles in newspapers and magazines, TV talk shows and series, films, the Internet, and even literary criticism. The cultural narratives of hysteria, which I call *hystories*, multiply rapidly and uncontrollably in the era of mass media, telecommunications, and e-mail.

As we approach our own millennium, the epidemics of hysterical disorders, imaginary illnesses, and hypnotically induced pseudomemories that have flooded the media seem to be reaching a high-water mark. These hystories are merging with the more generalized paranoias, religious revivals, and conspiracy theories that have always characterized American life, and the apocalyptic anxieties that always accompany the end of a century. Now they are dispersing globally to infect other countries and cultures.

I am a literary critic and a historian of medicine, rather than a psychiatrist. Above all, hysteria tells a story, and specialists in understanding and interpreting stories know ways to read it. As hysteria has moved from the clinic to the library, from the case study to the novel, from bodies to books, from page to stage and screen, it has developed its own prototypes, archetypes, and plots. Many of these motifs are adapted from myth, popular culture, folklore, media reports, and literature. Drawing on literary and medical history, I try to unravel some of the threads that make up the narratives of epidemic hysteria in the 1990s.

Hystories have internal similarities or evolve in similar directions as they're retold—which has convinced many doctors and researchers that these stories must be true. A century ago, Freud insisted that the stories his patients told him under hypnosis must be fact because of the "uniformity which they exhibit in certain details."[6] Dealing with chronic fatigue syndrome patients at the Centers for Disease Control in Atlanta, researcher Walter Gunn "asked himself the fundamental question: how could so many people—all of whom told a story that was, with only minor variations, the same—be making this up?"[7] Advocates of alien abduction also have faith in narrative similarity. "All the major accounts of abduction in the book share common characteristics and thus provide a confirmation of one another," writes David Jacobs in *Alien Encounters*. "Even the smallest details of the events were confirmed many times over. There was a chronology, structure, logic—the events made sense . . . and they displayed an extraordinary internal consistency."[8]

Literary critics, however, realize that similarities between two stories do not mean that they mirror a common reality or even that the writers have read each other's texts. Like all narratives, hystories have their own conventions, stereotypes, and structures. Writers inherit common themes, structures, characters, and images; critics call these common elements *intertextuality*. We need not assume that patients are either describing an organic disorder or else lying when they present similar narratives of symptoms. Instead, patients learn about diseases from the media, unconsciously develop the symptoms, and then attract media attention in an endless cycle. The human imagination is not infinite, and we are all bombarded by these plot lines every day. Inevitably, we all live out the social stories of our time.

The New Hysterians

While physicians and psychiatrists have long been writing obituaries for hysteria, scholars in the humanities and social sciences have given it new life. Social historians, philosophers, anthropologists, literary critics, and art historians have taken up the subject of hysteria because it cuts across historical periods and national boundaries, poses fundamental questions about gender and culture, and offers insights into language, narrative, and representation. This informal international network of scholars does not yet have an organization, a journal, or an official name, but we meet at conferences, correspond through e-mail and snail mail, and exchange manuscripts, articles, and books. I call the group the New Hysterians.

New Hysterians ask questions about the self, sexual and gender identity, cultural meaning, and political behavior. According to Roy Porter, a dauntingly prolific and energetic historian of medicine and science who teaches at the Wellcome Institute in London, the story of hysteria is "a history in which the very notions of mind and body, and the boundaries and bridges between them, are constantly being challenged and reconstituted."[9] In *Approaching Hysteria*, Mark Micale, who teaches at Yale and the University of Manchester, writes that hysteria is "not a disease; rather, it is an alternative physical, verbal, and gestural language, an iconic social communication."[10]

Throughout history, hysteria has served as a form of expression, a body language for people who otherwise might not be able to speak or even to admit what they feel. In the words of Robert M. Woolsey, hysteria is a "protolanguage," and its symptoms are "a code used by a patient to communicate a message which, for various reasons, cannot be verbalized."[11] It appears in the young as well as the old, in men as well as women, in blacks as well as whites. It happens to the powerful as well as the obscure. In October 1993, the Empress of Japan lost her voice after she had been criticized in the press and did not speak for three months: "It is possible," the official Japanese Household Agency declared, "for a person who suffers some strong feelings of distress to develop a symptom in which the person temporarily cannot utter words."[12] A seasoned soldier may experience stress as disabling as that of a helpless child. Circumstances silence people, not their rank or position.

Micale suggests that the new hysteria studies express the age as much as the disorders they analyze. He sees New Hysterians as products of the "gender revolution" inspired by the "great metacritique of

gender that in retrospect is certain to be regarded as one of the defining features of the thought, culture, and society of the late twentieth
century." He also speculates that this generation of scholars has come
of age in the context of the AIDS epidemic, reflecting "the rapid and
traumatizing reintroduction of the reality of epidemic disease" into
their mental life. Since mass psychogenic disorders are metasymbols
of the deep structures of our culture, Micale concludes that for the
New Hysterians, "rewriting the history of hysteria becomes a way of
achieving an understanding of, and perspective on, ourselves and our
social world."[13]

Beyond Scapegoats

I expect that defining recovered memory, chronic fatigue, and Gulf War
syndrome as contemporary hysterias, and analyzing them on a continuum with alien abduction stories and conspiracy theories will infuriate
thousands of people who believe they are suffering from unidentified
organic disorders or the aftereffects of trauma. I don't wish to offend
these sufferers, but I know that many assume the term *hysteria* has
insulting connotations. Being hysterical means being overemotional,
irresponsible, and feminine. During an argument, "hysterical" is what
you contemptuously call your opponent when you're keeping your
cool and he's losing his. It's a term that particularly enrages some feminists because for centuries it has been used to ridicule and trivialize
women's medical and political complaints.

Americans also tend to feel defensive about hysterical disorders
after the recent spate of accusations that this country is becoming a
hysterical victim society. It's a standing joke that Americans no longer
view themselves as sinners struggling with the guilt of lust, avarice, or
greed but rather as sick people addicted to sex, shopping, or sweets.
Books like Charles Sykes's *A Nation of Victims* (1992), Robert Hughes's
The Culture of Complaint (1993), Wendy Kaminer's *I'm Dysfunctional,
You're Dysfunctional* (1993), and Alan Dershowitz's *The Abuse Excuse*
(1995) mock and denounce what they see as the twelve-step, self-help
culture of contemporary America. Because many of these books have
an ideological ax to grind, they seek political scapegoats and simple
answers for a complex phenomenon. Pundits blame the recovery
movement on Freud and psychoanalysis, changes in sexuality, or a collapse of American family values. These attacks are so sweeping and so
vitriolic, so one-sided and so unfair, it's no wonder patients, psychia-

trists, and therapists feel threatened and panicky. In the *Journal of Psychohistory*, Nielltje Gedney, for example, charges that critics are after "the total annihilation of therapy and therapists."[14]

I don't regard hysteria as weakness, badness, feminine deceitfulness, or irresponsibility, but rather as a cultural symptom of anxiety and stress. The conflicts that produce hysterical symptoms are genuine and universal; hysterics are not liars and therapists are not villains. Instead, hystories are constructed by suffering patients, caring psychologists, dedicated clergy, devoted parents, hardworking police, concerned feminists, and anxious communities. While I criticize some forms of therapy, some uses of drugs in recovering memories, and some self-help literature, I also see a vital place for psychotherapy, psychopharmacology, and psychological guidebooks in everyday life. We should no more attempt to struggle alone with crippling depressions than to run the marathon with broken legs.

Unfortunately, though some critics claim that psychoanalysis is passé, Freud's message never got through to millions of people, who still distrust and fear the unconscious and its power over us. As a result, they suffer needlessly. Class, race, gender, and cultural attitudes play an underestimated role in the legitimation of psychotherapy. A 1995 *New York* magazine poll showed that 44 percent of New Yorkers living in Manhattan had sought psychological counseling—more than twice the percentage of those New Yorkers in Brooklyn, Staten Island, or Queens.[15] Black Americans distrust psychoanalysis more than white Americans do. Women have more leeway than men to seek psychological help.

Hysteria is inevitably a feminist issue, because for centuries doctors regarded it as a female reproductive disease. Charcot and Freud collaborated with female patients who have become known as the classical or canonical hysterics. Some modern psychoanalysts suggest that the golden age of hysteria vanished with the great hysterical divas of the nineteenth century. Jacques Lacan regarded these women as bygone stars, like Mistinguette or Judy Garland: "Where have they gone, the hysterics of yesteryear . . . these marvelous women, the Anna Os, the Emmy von Ns?"[16] he asked in 1977. But even in the 1990s, women patients outnumber men in virtually every category of unexplained illness and recovered memory. According to a study at Harvard Medical School, 80 percent of those with chronic fatigue syndrome are women. More than 90 percent of those who say they've recovered memories of childhood sexual abuse are women. Ian Hacking con-

cludes that nine out of ten patients diagnosed with multiple personality disorder are women. Researcher Debby Nathan observes that
accusations of satanic ritual abuse come primarily from women. Even
among those who claim to have been abducted by aliens, a field where
science fiction and technology mix, women outnumber men about
three to one and, according to ufologist David Jacobs, "seem to have a
larger number of more complex experiences."[17]

Hysteria concerns feminists because the label has always been used
to discredit women's political protest. Conservatives have pressed
ancient stereotypes into popular service to interpret all women's frustrations as sexual and irrational, and to stigmatize the sharing of
women's experiences as hysterical confession. Lynne V. Cheney's *Telling
the Truth* (1995), for instance, blames women's studies classrooms in universities for the recovered memory movement. Cheney draws a sinister
analogy between women's studies discussions and therapeutic coercion:
"Indeed, there are many parallels between the recovered memory
movement and feminism as it has come to be practiced on campuses.
The encouragement—even the requirement—in feminist classrooms
to confess personal views and traumas establishes an environment very
much like the one that exists in victim recovery groups."[18] Feminist
activists are understandably angry about these attacks and about related
attacks on the concepts of child abuse, date rape, and wife-battering.
They argue that these crimes are underreported and underbelieved,
that women and men have fought for years to create an atmosphere in
which women's testimony is taken seriously.

Nonetheless, in a surprising reversal, hysteria has been adopted
since 1970 by a number of feminist intellectuals, psychoanalysts, writers, and literary critics as a rallying cry for feminism itself. Some of
these women have claimed hysteria as the first step on the road to feminism, the sign of women's protest against patriarchy. Hysteria, writes
Diane Price Herndl, "has come to figure as a sort of rudimentary feminism, and feminism as a kind of articulate hysteria."[19] In my book *The
Female Malady* (1985), I speculated that although epidemic hysteria
exists on one extreme of a continuum with feminism, as a body language of women's rebellion against patriarchal oppression, it is a des-
perate, and ultimately self-destructive, form of protest. But for many
feminist writers, the nineteenth-century hysterical supermodels—the
canonical or articulate hysterics—epitomize universal female oppression. Some contemporary feminist theorists and therapists have inad-
vertently helped to spread new hysterical disorders.

The feminist interpretation of hysteria as a product of women's social circumstances has been an important contribution to our understanding of female psychology. But I deplore the credulous endorsements of recovered memory and satanic abuse that have become part of one wing of feminist thought. I try to ask feminist questions about the sources behind these syndromes, accusations, and conspiracy theories. What needs are women attempting to meet through these therapeutic investments, sickness lifestyles, and emotional hystories? Can we find more constructive ways to meet these needs than succumbing to the epidemic of suspicion and blame that threatens us all at the end of our century? Can we redefine hysteria in a way that allows more space for the mysteries of human emotions?

The Anatomy of Epidemics

In this book, I look at the forces that shape hysterical epidemics. Part I, "Histories," reviews the rise of modern hysteria and the cultural and religious matrix where it takes shape. Hysteria needs a doctor or theorist, an authority figure who can give it a compelling name and narrative. As Roy Porter points out, "The nineteenth century was hysteria's golden age because it was then that the moral presence of the doctor became normative as never before in regulating intimate lives."[20] The greatest of these physician-advocates were Jean-Martin Charcot, Sigmund Freud, and Jacques Lacan. But hysteria is dialogic: it depends on the needs of patients as well as the decisions of doctors. Until World War I, most of the famous hysterical patients were women. Many historians and analysts have maintained that hysteria is the product of a dialogue or collaboration between the hysterical woman and the medical man. Male doctors have been reluctant to confront the reality of male hysteria, but hysterical men play an underestimated role in the evolution of the disorder. I trace the theories and prototypes of male hysteria from the nineteenth century to the present and question the assumption that hysterical men must be homosexual.

In part II, "Cultures," I look at hysteria's intersections with literature, theater, and film. Models and metaphors of hysterical illness have always been circulated through fiction and drama, and Freud even defined hysteria as narrative incoherence. Today many syndromes are bracketed with a particular genre of popular fiction—multiple personality disorder with the confession, satanic ritual abuse with horror stories, alien abduction with science fiction. Movies and television also popularize the narratives of these syndromes, and even literary criticism can contribute to the blurring of fiction and reality.

Part III, "Epidemics," analyzes six psychogenic syndromes of the 1990s: chronic fatigue, Gulf War syndrome, multiple personality disorder, recovered memory of sexual abuse, satanic ritual abuse, and alien abduction. The hystories of these syndromes are linked and overlapping. Some doctors attribute Gulf War syndrome to chronic fatigue syndrome. Some therapists regard anorexia and bulimia as symptoms of childhood sexual abuse that must be remembered in therapy. Recovered memories of childhood sexual abuse can lead to cases of multiple personality disorder and satanic ritual abuse. Traumatologists believe that stories of alien abduction are screen memories for child sexual abuse, while ufologists maintain that narratives of child sexual abuse often shield experiences of alien abduction. All these syndromes move toward suspicion, conspiracy theories, witch-hunts, and mass panics.

Can we interrupt or halt these epidemics? I believe that we already have the power to control epidemic hysteria, though it will take dedication and persistence to counter sensational news reports, rumors, and fear. We must accept the interdependence between mind and body, and recognize hysterical syndromes as a universal psychopathology of everyday life before we can dismantle their stigmatizing mythologies. When anti-Freudian zealots make sweeping attacks on psychoanalysis and psychiatry, we can defend Freud's insights and try to restore confidence in serious psychotherapy. We need professional regulation that can establish licensing requirements for psychotherapists. We also need encouragement and financial support for people trying to cope with the painful dilemmas and tragedies of life in the 1990s. Psychiatry and pharmapsychology offer new and effective treatments for debilitating depression, compulsive behaviors, and anxiety disorders. TV talk shows and self-help literature are easy targets for scornful intellectuals, but they reach and teach a wide audience, largely female, that cannot always afford or manage other forms of counseling.

New Hysterians and other scholars can place hysteria in its fullest sexual, historical, and cultural contexts. We can use the media to fight rumors as well as to spread them, through op-ed pieces, magazine stories, TV documentaries, and books. Modern forms of individual and mass hysteria have much to tell us about the anxieties and fantasies of western culture, especially in the United States and Europe. We can use our knowledge of the past to interpret what is happening today. We can educate the public about the long history of war neurosis and transform the prevailing atmosphere of skepticism and contempt for psychogenic symptoms in men.

Feminists have an ethical as well as an intellectual responsibility to ask tough questions about the current narratives of illness, trauma, accusation, and conspiracy. We also have a responsibility to address the problems behind the epidemics—including the need to protect children from sexual and physical abuse. And we can lead the way in making distinctions between metaphors and realities, between therapeutic narratives and destructive hystories. If hysteria is a protolanguage rather than a disease, we must pay attention to what it is telling us.

Finally, as a critic of hysteria's stories, I want to emphasize my belief that hysteria is part of everyday life. Whenever I lecture about hysteria, I cough. French psychoanalyst André Green, an internationally honored member of the Freudian community, has joked that "we are all hysterics . . . except when we are writing papers." Any honest scholar knows that we are all hysterics, *especially* when we are writing papers. I do not have a quarrel with hysteria's symptoms, but with its social appropriations. In this book, I hope to show the difference.

2

Defining Hysteria

How do individual hysterias become social epidemics? How do these epidemics differ from mass hysteria? And how do hysterical epidemics or mass hysterias lead to witch-hunts?

What Is Hysteria?

Hysteria is not a single, consistent, unified affliction like malaria or tuberculosis. At first, as Dr. Philip Slavney of Johns Hopkins explains, hysteria "was regarded as a disease—an affliction of the body that troubles the mind." Later, the terms were reversed, and hysteria "was believed by many physicians to be an affliction of the mind that was expressed through a disturbance of the body," which converted unconscious desires into pathological changes and physical symptoms through an obscure neural process. Now hysteria "has come to imply behavior that produces the *appearance* of disease," although the patient is unconscious of the motives for feeling sick.[1]

Hysteria has been the designation for such a vast, shifting set of behaviors and symptoms—limps, paralyses, seizures, coughs, headaches, speech disturbances, depression, insomnia, exhaustion, eating disorders—that doctors have despaired of finding a single diagnosis. In 1878, a French physician, Charles Lasègue, proclaimed that "the definition of hysteria has never been given and never will be. The symptoms are not constant enough, nor sufficiently similar in form or equal in duration and intensity that one type, even descriptive, could comprise them all."[2] A century later, Edward Shorter lamented: "Writing a history of something so amorphous, whose meaning and content keep changing, is like trying to write a history of dirt."[3]

But another way into the history of hysteria is to see it as plural rather than singular, cyclical rather than linear—not, according to Roy Porter, "a single, unbroken narrative but scatters of occurrences: histories of hysterias."[4] Hysteria is a mimetic disorder; it mimics culturally permissible expressions of distress. An Englishman can legitimately complain of headache or fatigue but not that his penis is retracting into his body—a perfectly acceptable symptom in Malaysia and South China. Edward Shorter calls the legitimate symptoms in a given culture at a given time "the symptom pool." "By defining certain symptoms as illegitimate," he writes, "a culture strongly encourages patients not to develop them or to risk being thought 'undeserving' individuals with no real medical problems. Accordingly there is great pressure on the unconscious mind to produce only legitimate symptoms."[5]

A constant cultural negotiation goes on, of course, over both the symptom pool as a whole and the legitimacy of its contents. In the nineteenth century, Porter writes, the "visibility of real biomedical neurological disorders," like limps, paralyses and palsies, the result of birth defects, industrial accidents, alcoholism, venereal disease, and so on, provided "a sickness stylistics for expressing inner pains."[6] But many of these symptoms have declined or disappeared in the twentieth century and been replaced by new ones; the quantity of hysterical energy does not decrease but flows into new channels and takes new names.

Throughout most of its medical history, hysteria has been associated with women. Its name comes from *hystera*, the Greek word for uterus. Classical healers described a female disorder characterized by convulsive attacks, random pains, and sensations of choking. They believed the uterus traveled hungrily around the body, unfettered—Monday in the foot, Tuesday in the throat, Wednesday in the breast, and so on—producing a myriad of symptoms in its wake: a choking sensation, as if a ball were in the throat, called the *globus hystericus*; coughs and loss of voice; pains in various parts of the body; tics and twitches; paralyses, deafness, blindness; fits of crying; fainting; convulsive seizures; and sexual longings.

When anatomists proved that the uterus did not migrate, doctors relocated the centers of hysteria to the nervous system. Women were then described as a nervous sex, suffering from vapors, spleen, and fainting fits, or eroticized as hysterical nymphomaniacs. In fact, hysteria was often a wastebasket diagnosis. In his *Essay on the Pathology of the Brain* in 1684, Thomas Willis candidly acknowledged that hysteria was the term doctors used when they didn't know what they were seeing but wanted to say something: when "at any time a sickness happens in a Woman's Body, of an unusual manner, or more occult original, so that its causes lie hid, and a Curatory indication is altogether uncertain, . . . we declare it to be something hysterical . . . which oftentimes is only the subterfuge of ignorance."

By the eighteenth century blaming the nerves or the brain for hysterical symptoms also made it possible to recognize that men too might be sufferers, even though women still predominated as patients since they had fewer outlets for nervous energy (98 percent of the hysteria cases at Edinburgh Infirmary, for example, were female). As the English physician Henry Maudsley wrote in 1879, "The range of activity of women is so limited, and their available paths of work in life so few, compared with those which men have in the present social arrangements, that they have not, like men, vicarious outlets for feelings in a variety of healthy aims and pursuits."[7]

During the late eighteenth and early nineteenth centuries, some advanced physicians treated hysterical symptoms with mesmerism and animal magnetism, early experiments in hypnosis. Franz Anton Mesmer became a celebrity, demonstrating his techniques on French and Viennese ladies during the 1780s, when superstition contended with enlightenment rationalism. Mesmerism fell into disrepute by the middle of the nineteenth century, and hysteria remained a messy mystery. Although the number of hospital patients diagnosed as hysterical was small, the symptoms continued to fascinate doctors, who wrote about hysteria more than any other medical disorder. It also fascinated journalists, who quickly picked it up as a way of describing society. By 1900 hysteria had become widespread in the United States and Western Europe. Doctors explained the epidemic as a product of hereditary weakness and cultural degeneration.

Since Freud, psychology has sought an explanation for hysteria in theories of the volatile, histrionic personality; psychoanalysis has attributed it to Oedipal conflicts. Despite denials that hysteria is a female malady, questions of femininity are still central to psychoanalytic theory. The British psychoanalyst Gregorio Kohon has argued that all women go through a hysterical stage in their psychosexual development, during which they transfer their desires from the mother to the father. According to Kohon, "*A woman always at heart remains a hys-*

teric."[8] The French psychoanalyst Janine Chasseguet-Smirgel has hypothesized a female "aptitude for somatization." Women, she contends, turn emotions into physical manifestations because their sexuality is more diffuse than men's. Rather than being centered on a single visible organ, a woman's sexuality makes her entire body available for sexual symbolism.[9]

In recent years, hysteria has disappeared from consulting rooms, hospital wards, and psychiatric textbooks, as many of its traditional symptoms were reclassified as anxiety neuroses, obsessional disorders, manic depression, or borderline personality disorders. "In reality," wrote Georges Guillain, a French medical historian of hysteria, "the patients have not changed . . . but the terminology applied to them has."[10] What used to be called hysteria is now diagnosed as somatization disorder, conversion disorder, or dissociative identity disorder.

Despite this adoption of new terminology, many doctors and researchers feel that the concept of hysteria is still misleading, moralistic, and judgmental, either exaggerating the wisdom of the physician or trivializing the patient's pain. Richard Webster suggests that we might instead describe patients as suffering from "imaginary illness" and "imaginary symptoms," or postpone judgment altogether by calling them "unexplained physical symptoms." Perhaps, he adds, we should call the symptoms "spectral" rather than "imaginary," to give them more credence and weight.[11] While I recognize the difficulties of terminology, it makes sense to use the words *hysteria* and *hysterical*, both to draw on extensive records and to emphasize the continuities between past and present. Redefining hysteria as a universal human response to emotional conflict is a better course than evading, denying, or projecting its realities.

Modern Epidemics

Hysterical epidemics require at least three ingredients: physician-enthusiasts and theorists; unhappy, vulnerable patients; and supportive cultural environments. A doctor or other authority figure must first define, name, and publicize the disorder and then attract patients into its community. "Like invisible ink when heat is applied," writes Roy Porter, hysteria was "rendered visible by the medical presence."[12] The most influential doctors of hysteria are also theorists who offer a unified field theory of a vague syndrome, providing a clear and coherent explanation for its many confusing symptoms. Beginning with a small sample of patients, these doctors diagnose a puzzling disorder and give it a name. As Robert Aronowitz observes, the process works two ways; diagnosis is "an anticipated and necessary part of the healing ritual, bestowing a certain legitimacy on the patients' malaise, and at the same time undergirding the diagnostician's claim to social authority."[13] Doctors advocate a systematic method of treatment and hold out hope for a cure.

Influential diagnosticians have connections to institutions—clinics, hospitals, medical schools—which teach and promote their theories. The most famous and effective doctors have charismatic personalities and establish schools of devoted disciples. Interacting with modern media and culture, they become legends, caricatured in cartoons, satirized in drama, but also lionized in novels, plays, and movies.

Having diagnosed a new syndrome, physicians advertise prototypes of patients. For example, Gary Peterson, a psychiatrist who specializes in multiples, advises his followers to begin presentations with "a life course story." He provides them with a script about the life of a twenty-eight-year-old woman and urges them to "read the story slowly and emotionally, stopping at appropriate places to let the audience absorb the impact of what has just been said."[14] Self-help books also use real and composite prototypes to personalize a disorder. Like horoscopes, these prototypes are often broad enough to seem uncannily relevant. The media disseminate information about the prototype and encourage patients to come forward. Overall, clinical centers, professional newsletters and journals, and doctor-advocates increase a culture's investment in the syndrome as a real disease.

Yet no matter how persuasive the medical catalysts, hysterical epidemics would not erupt without the collaboration of patients. Edward Shorter writes that "hysteria offers a classic example of patients who present symptoms as the culture expects them or, better put, as the doctors expect them."[15] By the beginning of this century, some physicians had learned that hysteria could be *iatrogenic*—created by the interaction between doctor and patient. "It is not merely that his hypothesis is apt to color a physician's way of looking at a case," wrote the English doctor S. A. K. Wilson in 1901, "but also that in some obscure and little understood manner the patients come in a sense to respond to his hypothesis."[16] Cornell University historian Joan Jacobs Brumberg says the "interactive and evolving process" of a disease begins with social and cultural recruitment, as troubled individuals respond to prototypes.[17]

Initially, patients are people with a bewildering set of troubling symptoms and a wide range of explanations for them. Once they see their problems reflected in a prototype, come to believe that the laws of a disorder describe their lives, and seek the aid of a therapist, some patients rewrite their personal narratives. They may become addicted to their symptoms, and embark on the career of being a particular kind of patient, one with chronic fatigue syndrome, Gulf War syndrome, or multiple personality disorder. For some, the patient career may be a permanent way of life, with a self-supporting network of friends, activities, doctors, and treatments.

Many historians of psychiatry think the symbiotic relationship between male doctors and female patients explains the prevalence of women hysterics. In *The History of Sexuality*, Michel Foucault wrote that women have been made the passive, inert objects of a medical will to power. At the end of the nineteenth century, he wrote, women's bodies were "hystericized"—that is, turned into a collection of physical and psychological symptoms—by the medical profession. Henri Ellenberger, however, saw the relationships between young psychiatrists and hysterical female patients as more equal. These women tended to enter their physicians' lives at intellectually formative times in the doctors' careers, and they often served as clinical models—founding cases—of the doctors' theoretical work. The doctors needed hysterical women as muses; hysterical women needed doctors to speak for them.[18]

The third side of the hysterical triangle is environmental and cultural. Epidemics of hysteria seem to peak at the ends of centuries, when people are already alarmed about social change. The Salem witch trials took place in the 1690s; the mesmerism craze after the French Revolution, in the 1790s. In the 1890s, rebellions against imperialism and the class structure, controversies over prostitution and homosexuality, the rise of feminism, and the sexual plague of syphilis all joined with apocalyptic fantasies to produce the perception of a hysterical epidemic. In a supportive cultural environment, after entering the mainstream of popular culture, hysterical syndromes multiply as they interact with social forces such as religious beliefs, political agendas, and rumor panics. Traditional enemies or social scapegoats become part of the scenario, further fueling fears. The longer the epidemic continues, the greater the participants' need to believe it is genuine. In a sense, they feel their honor and integrity are at stake. The chain is hard to break, because each wave of publicity recruits new patients, who feel more and more invested in the search for an external cause and a "magic bullet" cure.

Anorexia and Bulimia

Anorexia and bulimia are examples of modern hysterical epidemics. Although anorexia nervosa was identified in 1874 and fasting behaviors had been observed for centuries before that, the rate of anorexia doubled between 1960 and 1976, and bulimia started its rise in the 1980s. By the late 1980s, these two disorders were thought to affect up to a million young women, and a U.S. House Subcommittee issued a report entitled "Eating Disorders: The Impact on Children and Families."

How did these epidemics occur? First, the cultural environment was supportive. American society from the 1960s on became increasingly obsessed with thinness, dieting, and exercise; anorexics seen in hospitals showed more severe weight loss than in earlier generations. Second, adolescent girls constituted a susceptible patient pool. And third, anorexia nervosa attracted a gifted physician-advocate who offered a coherent theory of the disease. Hilde Bruch, sometimes called "Lady Anorexia," was a professor of psychiatry at Baylor University Medical School in Houston, Texas. In two books, *Eating Disorders: Obesity, Anorexia Nervosa, and the Person Within* (1973) and *The Golden Cage: The Enigma of Anorexia* (1978), Bruch supplied a theoretical and sociological context for understanding food refusal. In her view, anorexia was about an adolescent's "struggle for control, for a sense of identity, competence and effectiveness," in a society that demanded slenderness, beauty, and obedience from its daughters. Bruch wrote compassionately about the anorexic's "paralyzing sense of ineffectiveness" and defined the prototype of the patient:

> The patients were described as having been outstandingly good and quiet children, obedient, clean, eager to please, helpful at home, precociously dependable, and excelling in school work. They were the pride and joy of their parents and great things were expected of them. The need for self-reliant independence, which confronts every adolescent, seemed to cause an insoluble conflict, after a childhood of robot-like obedience. They lack awareness of their own resources and do not rely on their feelings, thoughts, and bodily sensations.[19]

Often these adolescents had domineering mothers and equated eating with undesirable female sexual maturity.

Bruch's books humanized anorexia and, as Joan Jacobs Brumberg has explained, "provided an intimate account of the inner life of the anorectic." They connected anorexia to the "developmental crisis of adolescence," and "presented a nearly complete script" of the family tensions that provided the context for the disorder.[20] But even though *The Golden Cage* sold 150,000 copies and had a huge impact on young readers, medical books alone could not have created the epidemic. Beginning in the 1970s, the mass media circulated information about anorexia through news, articles in magazines like *Mademoiselle* and *Seventeen*, TV specials, movies, and best-selling novels.

Between 1980 and 1985, several anorexia autobiographies and celebrity revelations also came into the market. In 1983, when Jane Fonda revealed her problems with bulimia, girls who may not have known about vomiting as a form of weight control were exposed to the information. A decade later they could learn about bulimia through the tribulations of Princess Diana.

In young adult fiction, a set of narrative conventions described the inner world of an anorexic girl, and her eventual recovery. According to Brumberg, the plots were remarkably similar, even "formulaic," emphasizing "family tensions and the adolescent's desire for autonomy and control." The typical heroine is an attractive, ambitious high school girl, precisely five feet five inches tall, from a two-career family. "Like virtually all American girls, she embraces the current social ideal of slimness. . . . For various reasons all having to do with the difficulties of adolescence, ordinary dieting becomes transformed into a dominating pattern of ritualistic food and eating behavior."[21]

As these stories circulated, they put the blame for anorexia on the mother. Young adult novels about anorexia nervosa targeted the demanding, fashionable, often professional mother as the source of the heroine's conflicts about eating. "Because the main characters are depicted as still in high school and living at home," Brumberg explains, "mothers are central to the story. The fictive anorectic both dislikes and loves her mother and feels perpetually guilty about hurting and deceiving her." In fiction as well as reality, mothers rather than fathers seek out professional help for anorexic daughters. Despite their concern, mothers seem to be the daughters' antagonists across the dinner table.

By the late 1970s, through peer support groups, dormitory bull sessions, and college counseling, anorexia acquired a social life. Many of the eating disorder groups took a feminist position on the causes and contexts of the disorder, seeking to reduce the burden of individual or maternal responsibility by looking at social forces that demand thinness and passivity in women. At the same time, feminist writers and literary critics interpreted anorexia as a form of social protest, comparing it to the hunger strikes of imprisoned suffragettes and IRA terrorists. In *The Madwoman in the Attic* (1979), Sandra M. Gilbert and Susan Gubar described anorexia as a parodic or renunciatory gesture against patriarchal socialization. Other feminist critics speculated that Emily Brontë, Emily Dickinson, and Virginia Woolf may themselves have suffered from anorexia. Brumberg argued that anorexia nervosa has a spiritual dimension, that it substitutes for a code of meaning in the lives of young women: "Sadly, the cult of diet and exercise is the closest thing our secular society offers women in terms of a coherent philosophy of the self."[22]

As a result of all this attention, anorexia became epidemic. By the 1990s, some researchers recognized that publicity accorded to anorexia and bulimia was creating a secondary wave of patients, and that men too were developing eating disorders. The eating disorders unit at New York Hospital–Cornell Medical Center's Westchester Division admitted its first male patients in 1988. By 1995, men made up 13 percent of the cases.[23]

Mass Hysteria

A psychogenic epidemic like anorexia nervosa which develops and grows over a number of years is not the same as mass hysteria. When, because of panic and fear, people simultaneously contract physical or mental symptoms without any organic cause, that's mass hysteria. It's contagious; it spreads from one afflicted person to another but is usually abrupt and brief.

Mass hysteria has been recognized for centuries. In *Extraordinary Popular Delusions and the Madness of Crowds* (1841), Charles Mackay, a London journalist, described what he called "moral epidemics," including tulipomania and witchcraft. One hundred fifty years later, Mackay's book still has relevance. As Simon Wessely, a senior lecturer in psychological medicine at King's College School of Medicine in London, explains, "All that has changed is the precise nature of false explanation. In previous times mass hysteria would be blamed on demons, spiritism and diabolic possession. Nowadays we are oppressed by equally invisible gases, viruses and toxins." He points to such recent headline-grabbing phenomena as panics among Japanese commuters and shoppers following a poison gas attack on a Tokyo subway and nausea among children in Rhode Island, London, Osaka, the Palestinian West Bank, Albania, and Portsmouth.

Mass hysteria takes place within a community. According to Wessely, "The trigger is often trivial—one person has a heat-induced faint or a panic attack. Normally bystanders take little notice, but if the community is already in a state of tension a rumor can develop, usually 'we are being poisoned.' If the rumor is plausible to a wider group, it spreads rapidly." Witnessing someone else faint or collapse spreads the panic faster, and social networks sustain it. "If you do not know, or do not like, the person you see collapse in front of you, you are less likely to collapse. Hence outbreaks in tight-knit communities such as isolated villages or islands last the longest." Episodes are most severe when there is an obvious enemy; witness the Iraqi Scud missile attacks on Israel during the Gulf War, when some citizens believed they had been gassed and became nauseated or faint.

The reaction of authorities to these incidents and rumors is crucial. If ambulances arrive on the scene with sirens, if scare headlines ensue, and if a search for poisons takes precedence over calming fears, the situation rapidly gets out of control. "Things only go wrong," writes Wessely, "when the nature of an outbreak is not recognized, and a fruitless and expensive search for toxins, fumes, and gases begins. Anxiety, far from being reduced, increases. It is only then that long-term psychological problems may develop."[24]

Such episodes can affect men as well as women and children, health professionals as well as laymen. In February 1994 several emergency room workers in Riverside, California, fainted after treating a patient who vomited, went into cardiac arrest, and died. Although complications from cervical cancer caused the patient's death, hospital workers were convinced that they had been poisoned by a substance she emitted. The lawyer for one hospital worker objected to a report by the Department of Health that called the episode "an outbreak of mass sociogenic illness." "Clearly people were poisoned by something that night," he insisted. "These are all professional emergency room workers. They don't become hysterical because of a heart attack."[25] In January 1996 dozens of people in Canovanas, Puerto Rico, claimed to have seen a huge, vampirelike beast killing goats, sheep, rabbits, chickens, cats, and dogs. "It was about four or five feet tall and had huge elongated red eyes," said one witness. Although health authorities insisted that autopsies on the animals showed various causes of death, including parasites and feral dogs, panic about the monsters increased. Skeptics, according to the *New York Times*, recalled that "Puerto Ricans seem to have suffered almost cyclically from collective bouts of fear set off by sensationalist press accounts."[26] Soon after, the beast was spotted in Miami.

Witch-Hunts

When hysterical epidemics or mass hysterias target enemies, when they develop links with religious fundamentalism, political paranoia, or apocalyptic panic, they can turn into witch-hunts or pogroms. In his classic essay "The Paranoid Style in American Politics," historian Richard Hofstadter outlined millenarian paranoia, mass hysteria with a political form. Hofstadter wrote that while some paranoia may always be present in American politics, "movements employing the paranoid style are not constant but come in successive episodic waves," suggesting that "the paranoid disposition is mobilized into action chiefly by social conflicts that involve ultimate schemes of values and that bring fundamental fears and hatreds, rather than negotiable interests, into political action."[27]

Other scholars have argued that anxieties about social and economic change were relieved by attacks on witches. "Witchhunting," wrote Brian Levack, "became one of the ways that people could maintain their equilibrium at a time of great stress."[28] It guaranteed one's own sanctity and salvation despite theological and spiritual uncertainty. Norman Cohn described popular psychopathologies that attended the last millennium: many people "lived in a state of chronic and inescapable insecurity, harassed not only by their economic helplessness and vulnerability, but by the lack of the traditional social relationships on which, even at the worst of times, peasants had normally been able to depend. These were the people whose anxieties drove them to seek messianic leaders and they were also the people who were most prone to create demonic scapegoats." Mixed with old prophecies, wrote Cohn, paranoia "became a coherent social myth which was capable of taking entire possession of those who believed in it. It explained the suffering, it promised them recompense, it held their anxieties at bay, it gave them an illusion of security—even while it drove them, held together by a common enthusiasm, on a quest which was vain and often suicidal."[29]

Preconditions of a witch-hunt were consistent, whether the events took place in Scotland or Salem. The community had to know something about the practices of witches and to be convinced of their habits. Lawyers and judges also had to believe in witchcraft, since they controlled the judicial process and could halt the hunts. For successful prosecutions, specific antiwitchcraft legislation and the establishment of jurisdiction were necessary. Witch-hunts were smaller where inquisitional procedures and torture were prohibited, as in seventeenth-century England.

In addition, witch-hunts required an emotional atmosphere stirred up by sermons, discussions, and rumors. They often began with individual denunciations stemming from personal grudges. Sometimes malice played a role. Sometimes disturbed individuals confessed. In England, witch-hunts were usually limited to those originally accused. In Switzerland, Germany, and Scotland, medium-size witch-hunts, what Brian Levack calls "small panics," prevailed: the accused were tortured and implicated a group of accomplices. These panics burned themselves out when the local group of suspicious persons had been exhausted. As Levack remarks, "In communities where medium-sized hunts occurred, there may not have been a sufficient amount of popular hysteria for the less rigorous standards to be invoked."[30]

Large witch-hunts, "characterized by a high degree of panic or hysteria," took place in France, Sweden, and of course in Salem. These were driven by both the clinical conversion hysteria of the demoniacs and the collective hysteria of the community. Levack cautions that

we must be careful to distinguish between the mass hysteria of some witch-hunts and the individual psychological problems of some of the participants in these hunts. The occasional sadistic judge or hangman, the compulsive witch-finder, the insane or 'melancholic' witch all manifested abnormal forms of behaviour, but these should not be confused with the general, collective mood or group psychosis with which we are concerned. We must also be careful not to apply a simple label such as the 'witch-craze' or the 'witch-mania' or 'mass delusion' to the entire European witch-hunt. But within the context of specific witch-hunts we can legitimately—although at the same time hypothetically—talk about mass hysteria."[31]

In the notes to his prophetic play *The Crucible*, Arthur Miller explored the psychology and politics that created the Salem witch-hunt and, by extension, McCarthyism. Salem, Miller writes, "was a perverse manifestation of the panic which set in among all classes when the balance began to turn toward greater individual freedom." For some individuals it was a catalyst for repressed emotion, "a long-overdue opportunity for everyone so inclined to express publicly his guilt and sins, under the cover of accusations against the victims." It provided an opportunity to express "long-held hatreds of neighbors" and to take vengeance, "despite the Bible's charitable injunctions." The Salem witch-hunt began for political, social, and economic reasons; but it grew because "these people had no ritual for the washing-away of sins. It is another trait we inherited from them, and it has helped to discipline us as well as to breed hypocrisy among us."[32]

Cultures and Conspiracies

American culture has been particularly hospitable to hysterical movements. In the past, such movements have centered on the Masons, Catholicism, communism, the Kennedy assassination, and the fluoridation of water. In the 1990s, hysteria merges with a seething mix of paranoia, anxiety, and anger that comes out of the American crucible. Many observers see millennial America in the grip of what journalists Katherine Dunn and Jim Redden call "a mind-numbingly vast conspiracy theory."[33] *New Yorker* writer Michael Kelly terms this mix of conspiracy theories "fusion paranoia": "In its extreme form, paranoia is still the province of minority movements, but the ethos of minority movements—anti-establishmentarian protest, the politics of rage—has become so deeply ingrained in the larger political culture that the paranoid style has become the cohering idea of a broad coalition plurality that draws adherents from every point on the political spectrum."[34] These fantasies protect the real villains. Even a mother whose two little sons were killed in the bombing of the Federal building in Oklahoma City insists that the attack was part of a mysterious conspiracy: "Now I feel like I'm in some bad movie," she told a journalist. "Before this all happened, I never voted, never watched the news. Now I'm in the middle of a government conspiracy and cover-up. It just blows my mind."[35]

Some scholars warn that fusion paranoia has carried over to medicine and psychiatry, with conspiracy theories to explain every unidentified symptom and syndrome. Sherrill Mulhern, an outspoken American anthropologist who works in Paris at the wonderfully named Laboratoire des Rumeurs, des Mythes du Futur et des Sectes, sees a deeper problem behind the ostensible debate over memory: "the emergence of conspiracy theory as the nucleus of a consistent pattern of clinical interpretation. In the United States during the past decade, the clinical milieu has become the vortex of a growing, socially operant conspiratorial mentality, which is undermining crucial sectors of the mental health, criminal justice, and judicial systems."[36]

Americans may lead the world in these behaviors and attitudes, but other countries also provide breeding ground for hysterical epidemics. When Miller wrote *The Crucible* in the 1950s, he believed that "only England has held back before the temptations of contemporary diabolism," not only in religious tolerance, but in the absence of political persecution.[37] Even in the nineteenth century, British doctors believed that hysteria was rarer in the British Isles than elsewhere in Europe because of the sturdy and sensible quality of English culture and heredity. "The Gallic nature," wrote T. S. Dowse in 1889, "seems to be of less enduring stability than that of the Saxon, and is more liable to exhibit exalted hysterical manifestations."[38] "Certain races are more liable to the disease than others," wrote Edward Bramwell and John Tuke in 1910. "Thus the Latin races are much more prone to hysteria than are those who come of a Teutonic stock, and in more aggravated and complex forms."[39] In England doctors felt that hysteria was not only "un-English" but also un-Christian. As J. Mitchell Clark declared in *Hysteria and Neurasthenia*, "No race is exempt from hysteria, but it is more common in some than in others; thus the Jewish race is especially prone to suffer from it, and it appears to be more frequent, at any rate in a severe form, in France than in Germany or England."[40] While one hundred thirty-three book-length studies of hysteria were published in France between 1880 and 1900, England and Scotland together produced only four.

Today the English invariably reach for the metaphor of hysteria when they're confronted by political intensity or national drama. Hysteria is the opposite of the cherished national trait of irony. It is overstatement rather than understatement, wearing one's ambitions on one's sleeve, getting excessive, running it out. In English journalism, the term hysteria signifies disapproval of intensity, a put-down of both the antismoking lobby and the tobacco industry, of AIDS activists and homophobics, of feminists and misogynists.

In the 1990s, even the most cursory survey of the English press makes clear that too open a display of passion or ambition is regarded as hysterical. When John Major's sudden resignation as Tory Party leader in July 1995 led to a brief, ferocious public tussle among potential successors, the British press reacted with horror. A paradigmatic cartoon in *The Times* showed a staid John Major labeled "Englishman" and a rabid, foaming-at-the-mouth John Redwood (his Tory challenger) as "mad dog." In one essay, Simon Jenkins deplored the "hysterical talk" of "shell-shocked politicians": "The entire Tory party is engaged in a collective *crime passionnel*. If these are frigid Englishmen, Britain would be better run by a gang of mafiosi gigolos. We are at one of those alarming moments in our island story when someone (a Prime Minister, no less) peels back the skin of office to reveal, not a devotion to public duty or good government, but raw insecurity and ambition seething beneath."[41] The furor over Mad Cow Disease in 1996 owed some of its intensity to British fear and denial of anything mad.

On the other hand, at the Freud Museum's 1995 conference on "Hysteria Today," David Bell, a Kleinian analyst, observed that florid symptomatology of hysteria could still be seen in English psychiatric hospitals and that the full range of hysterical symptoms was far more common than many believed.[42] England has had its own outbreaks of hysterical panics over satanic ritual abuse, and Dr. Charles Shepherd estimated in 1992 that the country had one hundred thousand patients with chronic fatigue. English fiction and theater have taken the lead in exploring the meanings of hysteria for men and women today.

The French intellectual tradition of Cartesian hyper-rationality, skepticism, and anticlericalism has kept France relatively untouched by the more virulent recent panics. Sherrill Mulhern, a forceful critic of recent extremes, regards Paris as the perfect outpost from which to investigate flammable societies of hysteria. When it gets too hot in the brushfire conference circuit where recovered memory is debated, Mulhern can retreat to the relative academic safety of Neuilly and the cool intellectual detachment of her Parisian colleagues.

Nonetheless, France has a long hystory of its own. Throughout the twentieth century, while most psychiatrists have relegated hysteria to the dusty back shelves of the library, French doctors have showcased it under racy new titles, declared their affection for it, and pioneered its historiography. "When a foreign professor is asked to express his ideas in another country, he is expected to expose one of the most characteristic studies of his native land, just as, when we have landed in a new country, we seek to taste the dishes that characterize its cookery," said Dr. Pierre Janet in 1920 on the eve of his inaugural lectures at the Harvard Medical School. "It seems to me," he went on, "that what has been most characteristic in France for a number of years . . . is the development of pathological psychology," an interest that "has as its object a special disease: Hysteria."[43] Many French psychoanalysts still feel nostalgia for the heyday of hysteria and value national variants like *spasmophilie* that keep it alive.

Finally, even if contemporary hysterical epidemics begin in the United States, it was a nineteenth-century Parisian physician–enthusiast who pioneered the modern marketing of hysteria, who took it out of the medical books and made it a star. To understand modern hysterical epidemics, we must first look at Jean–Martin Charcot, and how he pioneered the synthesis of medical authority, institutional prestige, and cultural spectacle that initiated hysteria's golden age.

3

The History of Hysteria:
The Great Doctors

Jean-Martin Charcot:
The Invention of Modern Hysteria

The modern medical history of hysterical epidemics begins with Jean-Martin Charcot (1825–1893) and his clinic in the Paris hospital La Salpêtrière just over a century ago. Here doctor, patients, and culture came together for the first time. From the late 1870s until his death in 1893, Charcot, according to his student Axel Munthe, "was the most celebrated doctor of his time. Patients from all over the world flocked to his consulting-room in Faubourg St. Germain, often waiting for weeks before being admitted to the inner sanctum where he sat by the window at his huge library. . . . A word of recommendation from Charcot was enough to decide the result of any examination. . . . He ruled supreme over the whole faculty of medicine."[1] Magazines, newspapers, and fiction popularized Charcot's theories, and doctors from Europe and the United States sat at his feet. His French colleagues thought him the daring Caesar of hysteria. At the banquet for Charcot's election to the Institut de France, Professor Charles Bouchard said, "The study of hysteria could have brought you triumphant to Rome or dragged you into the mud. You were courageous and Fortune has rewarded your audacity."[2]

Charcot defined hysteria as a physical illness caused by a hereditary defect or traumatic wound in the central nervous system that gives rise to epileptiform attacks. His definitions and prototypes attracted thousands of clients; at the height of his power, approximately ten hysteri-cal women arrived at his clinic every day for diagnosis and treatment. Under Charcot's direction at the Salpêtrière, the percentage of women diagnosed with the disorder and hospitalized for it rose dramatically, from 1 percent in 1841 to 17 percent by 1883. In Paris, among the *char-coterie* of disciples and patients at the hospital, a particular kind of *grande hystérie* became epidemic; elsewhere, the syndrome was rare, leading some doctors to suspect that Charcot was creating iatrogenic illness or, indeed, inventing hysteria.

Charcot had extraordinary personal as well as intellectual gifts. He brought an artist's eye—the observational gift Freud would later term *visuel*—to the study of hysterical bodies. Many of his contemporaries described his mesmerizing gaze, and Dr. Alexandre Souques never for-got his "scrutinizing eyes . . . deeply set in the shadow of their orbits."[3] Charcot had planned to become an artist and always maintained a stu-dio in his home where he could paint. He and his interns sketched hysterical patients during their attacks, and he even installed a full pho-tographic studio, with a professional photographer, Albert Londe, to record the women's movements and expressions. These photographic images appeared in three volumes called *iconographies*; sketches, draw-ings, and paintings of the women were also reproduced and sold. The best known, André Brouillet's engraving of Charcot and his most famous hysterical patient, Blanche Wittman, hung in the lecture hall at the Salpêtrière, and Freud always had a copy in his office.

In the late 1870s Charcot, a showman with great theatrical flair, instituted two weekly public performances at the Salpêtrière. Every Friday morning, he gave a prepared lecture-demonstration, often involving hysterical patients. On Tuesdays, in the celebrated *leçons du mardi*, he publicly diagnosed patients he had never seen before—like a magician, or an acrobat working without a net. This bravado and vir-tuosity drew huge, spellbound audiences of as many as five hundred. Pierre Janet recalled, "Everything in his lectures was designed to attract attention and to captivate the audience by means of visual and audi-tory impressions."[4] According to Henri Ellenberger, "The podium was always decorated with pictures and anatomical schemata pertaining to the day's presentation. Charcot . . . entered promptly at ten o'clock, often accompanied by a distinguished foreign visitor and a group of assistants who sat down in the first row."[5] He illustrated his lectures with chalk drawings on the blackboard and imitated the behavior of patients he was about to present. Charcot certainly had a sense of the dramatic; on one occasion, when he planned to discuss tremors, he brought in three women wearing hats with long feathers, each of which trembled in a way characteristic of its disease.

Charcot undertook his studies at a propitious time. Because government ministers appointed medical directors at public hospitals, medicine and politics were intertwined. Political liberals and scientists shared anticlerical sentiments; Charcot explicitly set out to refute religion through his practice of medicine and, literary critic Martha Noel Evans asserts, to "reclaim hysteria from former religious interpretations of the disorder as diabolic possession, or, alternatively, saintly ecstasy."[6] He and his assistants wrote essays debunking miracles of the church, describing even Saint Joan of Arc as a case of hysteria. Paradoxically, however, Charcot himself used techniques that suggested the diabolism of the witch-hunt, such as searching for hysterical "stigmata" and pricking or writing on the sensitive skin of patients. In addition, Charcot's descriptions of hysterical seizures seemed influenced by religious imagery, and the epidemic hysterias at the Salpêtrière coincided with the reemergence of belief in miracles at the end of the century. In the late 1880s and early 1890s Charcot himself sent patients on a pilgrimage to Lourdes, and as Mark Micale points out, "Lourdes functioned as a kind of popular nonmedical counterculture of hysteria in late nineteenth-century Europe."[7]

Charcot had the advantage of working in a major medical institution, which he had redesigned in order to pursue his own interests. The Salpêtrière was a huge, old, rambling women's hospital in the 13th *arrondissement*, more poorhouse and medical warehouse than clinic. But even as an intern, Charcot saw in its thousands of long-term cases a living medical laboratory, a "reservoir of material," where he could test out theories through the "anatomical-clinical" method, performing autopsies for signs of organic disease and then tracing these signs back to their physical symptoms through close observation of patients. This old hospital was an ideal environment for the manufacture and marketing of hysterias, and Charcot made it an up-to-date "temple of science."[8] By the end of the nineteenth century, the Salpêtrière had become one of the sights of the city, a three-star attraction on any serious visitor's tour.

As chief physician at the Salpêtrière after 1862, Charcot made several important discoveries using the anatomical-clinical method. He differentiated multiple sclerosis from Parkinson's disease; defined the symptoms of poliomyelitis; mapped out the spinal forms of neurosyphilis; and described the pathology of amyotrophic lateral sclerosis, now called Lou Gehrig's disease.[9] In the 1870s, Charcot decided to use some of the same techniques to define the organic laws of hysteria. He theorized that hysteria was an inherited disease of the nervous system that could be triggered by an emotional or physical trauma in vulnerable men or women. Its symptoms ranged from stigmata, ovarian sensitivity, pain, visual disturbances, local numbness or anesthesias, particularly on the left side of the body, and convulsive fits. Charcot imposed a persuasive set of laws on the anarchic shapelessness and multiple symptoms—paralyses, muscle contractures, convulsions, and somnambulism—of hysteria. Furthermore, he set out to demonstrate that the dramatic seizures of *grande hystérie* could be induced or stopped by hypnosis, allowing doctors to examine its stages and determine its "laws." Jan Goldstein writes that he "took the old, amorphous 'wastepaper basket' of symptoms and replaced it with a coherent and conceptually elegant array."[10]

Though Charcot treated at least ninety male hysterics, about ten times that number of women were diagnosed as hysterics in the hospital. In his autopsies of hysterical women, Charcot concentrated on the ovaries—which, according to the reflex theories of medicine then popular, could send signals along the spinal cord to other organs. In examining patients, he found ovarian sensitivity, particularly on the left side, and began to use pressure on the ovaries to initiate and stop attacks. Soon he invented a physical apparatus, the ovarian compressor, a heavy leather and metal belt strapped onto the patient and often left for as long as three days. Later he would try to find parallel "hysterogenic" regions on men's bodies, compressing the testicles in an effort to affect the course of a seizure. (Unsurprisingly, the procedure did not always work, and some doctors discovered that squeezing the patient's testicles actually made the convulsions stronger.)

Charcot viewed seizures as the central sign of hysterical disorders. He outlined four stages: a premonitory period in which there might be visual disturbances or the classic *globus hystericus*; involuntary movements, building to backbending athletic acrobatics; stagy poses, which Charcot called *attitudes passionnelles* and suggestively titled "summons," "amorous supplication," "mockery," "menace," "eroticism," and "ecstasy"; and resolution. Predictably, he announced his unified theory of hysteria with dramatic panache and argued it with incontrovertible authority.

In 1878, Charcot reintroduced hypnosis, which had been discredited since the vogue for mesmerism and animal magnetism. He argued in

fact that the capacity to be hypnotized was itself a sign of hysteria. At
the Tuesday demonstrations in the hospital's semi-circular amphitheater,
women diagnosed as hysterics were put on display and hypnotized by
Charcot's interns. The Swedish doctor Axel Munthe recalled that one
woman "would crawl on all fours on the floor, barking furiously when
told she was a dog. . . . Another would walk with a top hat in her arms,
rocking it to and fro and kissing it tenderly when she was told it was her
baby."[11] Hypnotic suggestion was also used to stop hysterical attacks.
Charcot's theatrical demonstrations aroused controversies. Other doctors agreed that hypnotic suggestion was a powerful therapeutic tool but
disputed its special relationship to hysteria. Munthe complained, "If the
statement of the Salpêtrière school that only hysterical subjects were
hypnotizable was correct it would mean that at least eighty-five percent
of mankind was suffering from hysteria."[12]

Despite Charcot's insistence that hysteria was neither a sexual disorder nor one limited to women, both he and his staff repeatedly fell
back on stereotypes that equated it with the female personality.
Hysterics were seen as vain and preoccupied with their appearance,
deceitful and self-dramatizing. Charcot's assistant Charles Richet saw
these traits as "varieties of female character. . . . One might even say that
hysterics are more womanly than other women."[13]

At the Salpêtrière, two-thirds of the hysterical patients were working-class women. The nascent French feminist movement demanded
political, social, and educational reform but also provoked a backlash
of virulent misogyny. In addition, working women were neglected by
feminist thinkers and ignored—even betrayed—by the labor movement. Many working-class women migrated to the cities, where by
1866 they made up a third of the labor force. As Martha Noel Evans
comments, "Poor women were thrust into a new and often disorient-
ing freedom in urban centers. Alone, unsupported by the family
groups they were accustomed to, often paid below subsistence wages,
they faced a stressful lot. The astronomic increase in the number of
prostitutes in Paris at this time is a sad witness to the fate of many of
these displaced, young working women."[14]

Some of Charcot's working-class women patients became stars of his
public lectures and supermodels in his photography albums. Blanche
Wittman, known as the Queen of the Hysterics, and Augustine, later
the Surrealists' pinup girl, were among the most famous. Blanche
Wittman entered the Salpêtrière in 1877 at the age of fifteen. The
daughter of a carpenter who had himself been institutionalized, she had

worked as a laundress, a furrier's apprentice, and a nurse. Her symptoms of convulsions and "nervous crises" began when the furrier attempted to rape her. In the Salpêtrière, Wittman proved to be an excellent hypnotic subject; George Frederick Drinka writes in *The Birth of Neurosis* that her "astonishing cataleptic, lethargic, and somnambulistic feats were reported in detail throughout the Western medical world."[15] Painted, displayed, and photographed, she stayed in the hospital for her entire life. After Charcot's death she became a laboratory technician and eventually a radiologist. Even on her death bed she insisted that her fits had been genuine.

Augustine spent only five years in the Salpêtrière, from October 1875, when she was a fifteen-year-old domestic servant, to September 1880; but she became the most photographed of all the hysterical patients. At age thirteen, she had been raped by her mother's lover, who had threatened her with a knife; soon after, she began to have seizures in which she imagined that she was being bitten by wild dogs or rats and chased by a knife-wielding man. In the hospital, she was treated with drugs, straitjackets, and solitary confinement as well as hypnosis, and posed frequently for Londe. After many attempts to run away, she finally succeeded by disguising herself as a man.

Charcot's images of the hypnotized hysterical woman inspired novels and plays, which in their turn influenced popular understanding of the hysterical trance. In the 1880s, art students who had been to performances at the Salpêtrière amused themselves by hypnotizing their models. "The chief culprit," wrote one contemporary, "was a young fellow who for some considerable time had attended the lectures of the late Dr. Charcot, and, rather than waste the knowledge he had acquired, he applied it indiscriminately to no matter whom—models and fellow-workers alike. . . . Our amateur Charcot continued to experimentalize, and finally selected for his "subject" a girl of great plastic beauty; . . . the well-known Elise Duval, the favorite model of MM. Gérôme and Benjamin Constant. . . . One day at the beginning of a seance, she was thrown into a trance which lasted for four hours, at the end of which time she was awakened more dead than alive." The atelier of Gérôme was closed for a month over the scandal.[16]

The idea of the vulnerable artist's model entering a trance in order to pose for hours resurfaced in George Du Maurier's best-selling novel *Trilby* (1894), which became a great hit play of the fin-de-siècle stage. The young artist's model Trilby suffers from crippling migraine headaches; she is cured by the mesmerism of the Jewish musician

Svengali, under whose hypnotic gaze and instruction she becomes a great singer. *Trilby* sold over two hundred thousand copies in its first year and generated a craze—"Trilby-mania"—for sequels and spin-offs. The stage and film versions played up Svengali's Jewishness and further demonized the mesmerist; Trilby became a popular icon of hysterical suggestibility and feminine attractiveness.

Even in Charcot's day, these theatrical poses and fictional heroines taught women how hysterics looked. The performances took place in a hall of mirrors, for the hysterics were coached and surrounded by pictures of *grande hystérie*. Some of the women in the Salpêtrière acquired symptoms related to the photography itself; a sixteen-year-old seamstress, Hortense, came down with "photophobia," a spasm and paralysis in one eye induced by the flash—a squint that made her face mimic that of the cameraman.[17] Charcot's favorite model, Augustine, had episodes of color blindness when she saw everything in black and white. Indeed, as Jan Goldstein has concluded, "The 'iconography' of hysteria as defined by Charcot—with all its vividly theatrical contortions and grimaces—seems to have been so widely publicized . . . in both pictorial and verbal form, as to constitute for that historical moment a reigning 'cultural preconception' of how to act when insane."[18]

Despite his brilliance, Charcot made a number of mistakes. According to Henri Ellenberger, he wrongly emphasized the most complex forms of hysteria and oversimplified the disease descriptions to make them fit into his scheme. He was not interested in his patients as people; he cared about them only as cases. "Charcot hardly ever made clinical rounds himself; rather, he saw his patients in the hospital examining room while his students, who had examined them in the wards, reported to him. Charcot never suspected that his patients were often visited and magnetized repeatedly on the wards by incompetent people."[19] The Goncourt brothers reported in their diary that Charcot gossiped about patients' personal secrets.

Having started with the intention of making objective scientific discoveries about hysteria, Charcot ended with a rigid model, a theoretical cage into which he squeezed all his patients. In the highly contagious environment of the hospital, hysteria took on the immense power of suggestion. People came in with problems—with psychosomatic conversion symptoms, post-traumatic stress disorders, and other emotional responses to their unhappy lives. Charcot gave them a diagnosis; he gave them a certain degree of legitimacy; he even gave some of them a warped celebrity. But he took away their dignity and their hope. They were pressed into mass conformity, put into solitary confinement, turned into chronic, even lifelong patients. Through hypnotic suggestion, Evans notes, "hysterical patients were already becoming iatrogenic monsters."[20]

Toward the end of his life, Charcot suspected that his theories were flawed and that he needed to pay more attention to the psychological and social elements in his patients' lives. Moreover, the liberal political atmosphere in France that had supported his work was shifting to the right in the early 1890s. After his death in 1893, Charcot's fame rapidly declined. As Mark Micale writes, the empire of hysteria that had made France "for a single, glorious generation . . . the international epicenter of the hysteria industry" began to "break apart" and "scatter."[21] Charcot's medical rivals, such as Hippolyte Bernheim in Nancy, challenged his theories, and some of his own interns suggested that he had coached his patients in their performances. In his savage novel *Les Morticoles* (1894), Léon Daudet portrayed Charcot as the sinister Doctor Foutange, who manipulates his patients like a puppeteer. Swiss neurologist Paul Dubois noted that in the Salpêtrière, "All cases of hysteria resemble each other. At the command of the chief of the staff, or of the interns, they begin to act like marionettes, or like circus horses accustomed to repeat the same evolutions."[22]

By 1900, writes Micale, "the age of Charcot, and with it the *belle époque* of French hysteria, had effectively come to a close," and a backlash against his theories had set in.[23] A German doctor predicted that "within a few years the concept of hysteria will belong to history." What Charcot had called hysteria, he claimed, was "a tissue woven of a thousand threads, a cohort of the most varied diseases, with nothing in common but the so-called stigmata, which in fact may accompany any disease."[24] A year later, Charcot's former pupil Joseph Babinski presided over a meeting of the Paris Neurological Society that systematically dismantled all the assumptions of the Charcotian model of hysteria. In an article for a medical journal, Babinski announced the "dismemberment of traditional hysteria."[25] By the 1930s, only one dissertation on hysterical disorders was written at French medical schools.[26]

Sigmund Freud: The Talking Cure

Charcot had publicized the idea of hysteria as a unified organic disease; Sigmund Freud, who had studied at the Salpêtrière in 1885 and 1886, defined it as a neurosis caused by repression, conflicted sexuality,

and fantasy. Freud felt that the course of his intellectual and professional life had been changed by his encounter with Charcot, who was
brilliant, cultivated, and bold in his thinking, with an extraordinary
ability to encapsulate and theorize. Among Charcot's many admirers
and disciples, only Freud had the charisma and determination to build
a theoretical empire. Indeed, Richard Webster contends, "Freud himself consciously identified with Moses, and the prophetic and messianic dimensions of his character."[27]

Like Charcot, Freud was a showman who publicized psychoanalysis through his writings and lectures. Although Charcot worked with,
and perhaps created, the florid behaviors of *grande hystérie*, Freud
worked with the much more subtle, everyday symptoms of *petite hystérie*: coughs, limps, headaches, loss of voice—conversion hysterias with
less dramatic potential. In the 1890s, when Charcot's career had
reached its apex and Freud's was on the rise, hysteria coincided with
the unconscious anxieties and fantasies of the fin de siècle to produce
a powerful mix unequaled until the end of our own century. Freud's
ideas on hysteria are scattered throughout his writing, but they peak in
the 1890s, when, as John Forrester and Lisa Appignanesi point out,
they became "grand theories, colossal structures, breathtaking specula-
tive leaps."[28] These ideas are fundamental to our century's way of
thinking about hysteria.

Along with his colleague Joseph Breuer, Freud took the crucial step
of actually listening to hysterical women and paying serious attention
to their stories. In the lengthy *Studies on Hysteria* (1895), Freud and
Breuer proposed a new explanation for the origin of hysteria and a
new therapy for its treatment, arguing that all hysteria, male and female,
had traumatic origins, but that the traumas did not have to be injuries
or hereditary lesions. Instead, they could be disturbing sexual experiences patients had repressed, thus creating symptoms through a process
of symbolization. The original traumatic injuries, they speculated, had
occurred when the patient was in a "hypnoid state," moments of day-
dreaming or resistance to pain. The memories were then banned from
consciousness and converted into bodily symptoms that were
"mnemonic symbols" or physical metaphors of the suppressed trauma.
If the patient could retrieve these memories through hypnosis, along
with their original force or affect, her symptoms would vanish.

In 1880, Breuer thought he had relieved the symptoms of his first
patient, Bertha Pappenheim (1859–1936), whom he named "Anna O.,"
through the process of hypnosis and analysis she called "the talking

cure." Breuer described Anna O. as "markedly intelligent, with an astonishingly quick grasp of things and penetrating intuition. She possessed a powerful intellect which would have been capable of digesting solid mental pabulum, and which stood in need of it." Although she was "bubbling over with intellectual vitality," Anna O. "led an extremely monotonous existence in her puritanically-minded family." Her hysterical conversion symptoms—including a severe cough, headaches, contractures of her right arm and leg, sleepwalking, and loss of voice—seemed in part an expression of intellectual frustration. In lengthy sessions Breuer invited her to speak, often under hypnosis, about her memories, dreams, and hopes. This attention seemed to help, but the therapy ended abruptly when Anna O. hallucinated that she was giving birth to Breuer's baby. She had also become addicted to pain-relieving drugs and spent several months in sanatoriums between 1883 and 1887. In the 1890s, Pappenheim worked with Jewish immigrants from Eastern Europe and found a satisfying outlet for her talents in feminist journalism, politics, and philanthropy.[29]

In his early work with hysterics, Freud used techniques he had learned from his teachers, especially Charcot. He attempted to provoke hysteria by pressing the "hysterogenic" ovarian zones of his women patients' bodies. And like Breuer, he used hypnosis to help patients recall early childhood memories he believed had been forgotten or repressed. This technique, the "cathartic method," he later explained, differed from hypnotic suggestion and involved "questioning the patient upon the origin of his symptoms, which in his waking state he could only describe very imperfectly or not at all."[30] Like theorists of neurasthenia, Freud blamed masturbation for such symptoms as fatigue, constipation, and bed-wetting. For a decade, influenced by the theories of an eccentric friend, the Berlin doctor Wilhelm Fliess, he even believed that sexual problems had their source in the nose.

Freud hypothesized that the doctor must insist on taking memories back to their sources in order to bring about a cure. Treating twenty-seven-year-old Emma Eckstein for vague complaints, including stomach aches and menstrual irregularities, in 1895, Freud initially concluded that her hysteria was caused by masturbation and the cure was to operate on her nose. Fliess performed the operation but bungled it, leaving a piece of gauze in the nasal cavity that caused a severe postoperative infection. Meanwhile, Freud had convinced himself that Emma's postoperative symptoms and hemorrhages were merely hysterical manifestations. When discussions of her childhood masturbation did not help,

Freud urged Emma to come up with other "memories"—an account of sexual abuse when she was eight, and even a story about satanic ritual female circumcision.

By 1896, Freud was convinced that repressed childhood or even infantile sexual abuse caused hysteria; he called this early model of hysteria the seduction theory. In a paper read to the Viennese Society for Psychiatry and Neurology in April 1896, based on his experiences with eighteen hysterical patients, Freud announced his views on the etiology of hysteria. "At the bottom of every case of hysteria," he said, "there are *one or more occurrences of premature sexual experience*, occurrences which belong to the earliest years of childhood but which can be reproduced through the work of psycho-analysis in spite of the intervening decades." Hysterical symptoms were the "derivatives of memories which are operating unconsciously." As he wrote to Fliess in December 1896, he had come to believe that in most cases the fathers were the seducers and abusers. "It seems to me more and more that the essential point of hysteria is that it results from *perversion* on the part of the seducer, and *more and more* that heredity is seduction by the father."[31]

But unlike Charcot, who died before he could revise his own too sweeping and too simple theory of hysteria, Freud moved through several stages. By late 1897, he had abandoned the seduction theory for a concept that depended much more on the patient's unconscious and on sexual and Oedipal fantasy. Freud announced his new theory in another letter to Fliess, listing the reasons he had been forced to abandon his seduction hypothesis. First, the theory did not lead to therapeutic success. Second, the incidence of fathers abusing children would be improbably vast, because it would have to exceed the incidence of hysteria. Third, no one could distinguish between truth and fantasy in narratives elicited from the unconscious. And finally memories of abuse never surfaced except when his patients were under hypnosis, "even in the most confused delirium." Therefore, Freud concluded, instead of remembering real incidents of incestuous abuse, hysterical patients were expressing fantasies based on their unconscious Oedipal desires.

Freud's abandonment of the seduction theory has long been the center of heated debate about hysteria, psychoanalysis, and the character of Freud as a man. In 1980, as he recalls in *The Assault on Truth: Freud's Suppression of the Seduction Theory* (1984), psychoanalyst Jeffrey M. Masson, then projects director of the Freud Archives, "was given the freedom of Maresfield Gardens, where Freud spent the last year of his life. Freud's magnificent personal library was there, and many of the volumes, especially from the early years, were annotated by Freud."[32] Masson made several discoveries, including letters about the sexual seduction of children, and a pattern of omitting such discussions in Anna Freud's abridged edition of the Freud/Fliess letters. Masson pursued the issue of a cover-up, and in August 1981 the *New York Times* reported his discoveries, leading to a furor in which he was dismissed from the Freud Archives.

The furor over Freud, however, has never really subsided. Freud was a fraud, some angry feminists charged. For Freud "to incriminate daughters rather than fathers," wrote Judith Lewis Herman in *Father-Daughter Incest* (1981), "was an immense relief to him, even if it entailed a public admission that he had been mistaken." Freud, she protested, all but forgot the incestuous wishes of parents in his new zeal, which did not "matter very much in the case of boys, for, as it turns out, boys are rarely molested by their parents. It matters a great deal in the case of girls, who are the chief victims."[33]

Masson declared that in publicly renouncing his seduction theory, Freud backed away from the true complaints of his women patients and that he did so out of self-exculpation and professional cowardice. "By shifting the emphasis from an actual world of sadness, misery, and cruelty," Masson wrote, "to an internal stage on which actors performed invented dramas for an invisible audience, Freud began a trend away from the real world that, it seems to me, is at the root of the present-day sterility of psychoanalysis and psychiatry throughout the world."[34]

But many other recent critics of Freud, including Allen Esterson, Morton Schatzman, Frederick Crews, and Richard Webster, argue persuasively that Freud pressured his patients to produce narratives congruent with his theories. In other words, Freud's patients were not molested by their fathers and did not fantasize about them. Instead, they fabricated stories along the lines of Freud's own hysterical hypotheses. "Before they come for analysis," Freud himself admitted in "The Aetiology of Hysteria," "the patients know nothing about these scenes." Their "memories" of abuse were responses to Freud's hints, suggestions, and persuasion. Indeed, Freud wrote that he preferred a method of diagnosing the causes of hysteria "in which we should feel less dependent on the assertions of the patients themselves." When the patient's memories did not satisfy the therapist's expectations of traumatic causation, Freud explained, "We tell our patient that this experience explains nothing, but that behind it there must be hidden a more significant, earlier experience; and we direct his attention by the same technique to the associative thread which connects the two memories—the one that has been discovered and the one that has still to be discovered."

Clearly, Freud was a stubborn, bullying interrogator of hysterical women. In *Studies on Hysteria*, he explained how the therapist must fight to overcome the patients' defenses: "We force our way into the internal strata, overcoming resistances all the time." By March 1896, Freud argued that the stories must be true *because* the patients were not conscious of remembering them and stammered or cried while describing them under hypnosis. A month later, he defended himself against the idea that "the doctor forces reminiscences of this sort on the patient" by pointing to the "uniformity" of the narratives.[35]

Looking closely at Freud's letters and essays from this time, I am convinced that he did force such reminiscences on his patients, eliciting confabulations rather than actual memories. As Berkeley professor Frederick Crews puts it, "Freud himself laid down the outlines of the seduction plots, which were then fleshed out from 'clues' supplied by his bewildered and frightened patients, whose signs of distress he took to be proof that his constructions were correct."[36] Richard Webster endorses this view and adds that renouncing the seduction theory moved Freud further away from hypotheses based on evidence: "What happened when Freud repudiated his seduction theory, then, was not that he abandoned the real world of human emotions for an invisible world of internal biological processes. . . . What happened was that this invisible world was at last almost completely freed from the constraints of empirical reality."[37]

We see effects of this shift to internal, invisible dramas in Freud's case study of Ida Bauer, or "Dora," whom he treated in 1900. Brought to Freud's Vienna consulting room by her father when she was eighteen, Dora was an intelligent young Jewish woman stifled by the limitations of her role as the marriageable daughter of a bourgeois family. She was a Viennese version of the New Woman of the 1890s, the feminist who seeks higher education and wishes to avoid marriage, but she was also dealing with the rising anti-Semitism of Austrian society. Freud never met Dora's mother, whom he regarded as an obsessive housewife. Although Dora felt contempt for her mother's monotonous domestic life, it was the life for which she too was destined. Her mother was "bent upon drawing her into taking a share in the work of the house." Dora could find no support for her intellectual aspirations from either parent. Although she had a governess who was "well-read and of advanced views," Dora believed that the governess was neglecting her and was really in love with her father. She arranged to have the woman dismissed. Afterward, she struggled alone with the effort to keep up her serious reading, and she attended lectures specially given for women. Her older brother, Otto, went off to the university and later became a prominent Austrian politician.

Dora was treated like a pawn or a possession by her father and denied the rights to privacy or personal freedom. For six years her father had been having an affair with Frau K., whose husband had attempted to seduce Dora when she was fourteen. Dora felt that "her father had handed her over to Herr K." in exchange for his complicity in the adultery. Professing to be anxious about her depressive state of mind but really, Dora believed, afraid that she would betray his sexual secrets, her father then "handed her over" to Freud for psychotherapeutic treatment. He wanted Freud to persuade Dora that her keen perceptions were simply adolescent imaginings. He hired Freud hoping for an advocate to "bring her to reason."[38]

As Jeffrey Masson observes, Dora had good reason to be upset: "She felt conspired against. She was conspired against. She felt lied to. She was lied to. She felt used. She was used."[39] Freud's determination to label her as a hysteric did not depend upon the severity of her symptoms, which were few and slight; she had a chronic cough, headaches, depressions. Although he acknowledged that Dora's case was no more than *petite hystérie*, Freud believed that the ordinariness of her symptoms made her an ideal psychoanalytic subject. Committed from the start to the hysteria diagnosis, he interpreted all Dora's behavior and statements in accordance with his theories. He told her that she was really attracted to Herr K., in love with her father, and with Freud himself. He ignored the appalling circumstances of Dora's family situation, and after only eleven weeks she broke off the therapy.

Unlike the impoverished working-class women at the Salpêtrière, who had to give Charcot what he wanted, Dora had the financial and social resources to resist her therapist. Yet Dora failed as well. She was not a willing participant and did not collude with Freud, but she couldn't manage to tell her own story. Instead, Freud used her to publicize psychoanalysis at the moment of its inception and rising fortunes. Freud's account, called "Fragment of an Analysis of a Case of Hysteria," was published in 1905 and has become the most famous study of any hysteric.

Analysts today believe that psychoanalysis could only have evolved out of work with hysterics because hysterics formed strong, explicit transferences to their doctors and thus provided examples of projection and sexual conflict. Kurt Eissler has hypothesized that "the discovery of psychoanalysis would have been greatly impeded, delayed, or even made impossible if in the second half of the nineteenth century the prevailing neurosis had not been hysteria."[40] "I think . . . that psychoanalysis had to start from the understanding of hysteria," Juliet Mitchell writes. "It could not have developed from one of the other neuroses or psychoses. Hysteria led Freud to what is universal in psychic construction and it led him there in a particular way—by route of a prolonged and central preoccupation with the difference between the sexes. . . . The question of sexual difference—femininity and masculinity—was built into the very structure of the illness."[41] However, Freud relied on cultural myths of masculine and feminine identity in shaping his interpretation of hysteria. Had he written a case study of "Dorian" rather than "Dora," the history of psychoanalysis might look very different.

On the whole, Freudians make strict distinctions between hysterical symptoms and psychosomatic symptoms. Hysteria, Martha Noel Evans sums up, is "primarily a pathological personality structure resulting from inner psychic conflict."[42] The conversion symptom of hysteria is a particular form of symbolic somatization; it represents a transfer of libido to a bodily organ that expresses a forbidden wish and its feared consequences. Freudians view paralysis in a leg, without organic cause, as a hysterical symptom, both an erection and a castration, while hysterical blindness is both a wish to look at something forbidden and the punishment for such transgression. Migraine headache or stomach pain, however, might be merely somatic and have no symbolic content. How psychiatrists tell the difference between hysterical and psychosomatic symptoms is hard for a layman to figure out, but as a result of this distinction hysteria has been severed from ordinary experience. Everyone admits to having the occasional psychosomatic episode. But rather than explaining hysteria as a point further along a spectrum of universal human behavior, psychoanalysis has made it seem aberrant and enigmatic.

As we approach the second century of Freudian studies, the Freudian empire seems to be collapsing, just as Charcot's empire did a century ago. While Freud was long the subject of hagiography, he is now the subject or object of pathography, as biographers vie with one another to produce the most demonic and maniacal life history. In a 1993 essay called "The Unknown Freud," which appeared in the *New York Review of Books*, Frederick Crews, who began his career as a psychoanalytic literary critic, denounces Freud as "willful and opportunistic," and calls psychoanalysis so scientifically feeble that it could be sustained only "in popular lore, the arts, and the academic humanities, three arenas in which flawed but once modish ideas, secure from the menace of rigorous testing, can be kept indefinitely in play."[43] British literature professor Richard Webster goes even further: in *Why Freud Was Wrong* (1995), Webster denounces Freud as a man with a Jewish Messiah complex who ruthlessly twisted the facts and sacrificed his patients.

Both Crews and Webster hold Freud responsible for the recovered memory movement, which they deplore. In the fall of 1995, Freud's critics protested so vociferously against the Library of Congress's planned Freud exhibition that it was indefinitely postponed. The exhibit, Crews charged, was "conceived as a means of mobilizing support for the besieged practice of psychoanalysis."[44] Even as psychoanalysts celebrated the centenary of Freud and Breuer's *Studies on Hysteria* in 1995, Freud bashing reached a peak of frenzy. Some predicted that like Marxism, psychoanalysis was an ideology that could not survive the millennium.

Of course, some intellectuals have always scoffed at Freud. But Crews, Webster, Masson & co. offer little to replace his insights or vision. Webster argues that virtually all psychological symptoms are organic, and that every case of hysteria has been misdiagnosed. Crews enjoys the traditional position of the critic, who does not have to do more than attack. Whatever the assaults of academics and renegades, artists and writers will continue to cherish Freudian insights. The British novelist Sebastian Faulks comments, "Most people have a Freud-shaped cavity in their minds which no other writer can satisfactorily fill. The climate of opinion he created will take an age to alter. He offers intellectual excitement, literary pleasure, magical solutions, and all in the cause of healing humankind. One would as soon discard God or Santa Claus."[45] Despite his mistakes, Freud in my view was a truth seeker, willing to revise his ideas and to criticize himself. The therapy he pioneered has changed drastically since the days when he treated hysterics in Vienna, and Freud would probably not recognize or even endorse some of its current forms. Yet at its heart and at its best, psychotherapy offers a safe space within which we can examine the most frightening, damning, and forbidden parts of ourselves, and come to take responsibility for our future.

Jacques Lacan

Since Freud's death in 1939, the strongest contender for the position of hysterical impresario has been Jacques Lacan (1901–1981), who founded the École Freudienne de Paris in 1964. In his rereadings of Freud with a structuralist/poststructuralist twist, Lacan became a French Freud who interpreted hysteria as a linguistic and cultural phenomenon and a metaphor for Woman and femininity. Like the 1880s in Paris and the 1890s in Vienna, Paris in the 1970s and 1980s was a hospitable milieu for psychoanalytic gurus and theories of hysteria. In her important book *Psychoanalytic Politics*, MIT professor Sherry Turkle examines the ways psychoanalysis displaced and assimilated Marxism and other radical political movements after the collapse of the 1968 student revolution. Disappointed intellectuals turned from political action to philosophical inquiry.

"Since 1968," Turkle writes, "a Frenchman often finds a psychoanalyst in places where he might once have expected to find a priest, a teacher, or a physician. Analysts lived through the May–June events to find that by the time the dust had settled, they were no longer marginal men and women but were very much at the center of things. For many people, psychoanalysis, which was once seen as subversive and alien, was now a welcome source of expertise for solving the problems of everyday life."[46] According to his biographer Elisabeth Roudinesco, Lacan was leader and savior for a generation: "like Charcot at the Salpêtrière and like Freud in Viennese society, Lacan, as of 1969, became the iconoclastic doctor of a society sick with its symptoms, its mores, and its modernity."[47]

Many of Lacan's critics and disciples have remarked on his similarity to Charcot; Martha Noel Evans writes, "Not since the clinical lessons of Charcot a century earlier had a master of French medicine exercised the same kind of influence and charisma as Jacques Lacan."[48] Like Charcot, Lacan was a dazzling theoretician, a charismatic and iconoclastic clinician, an aesthete with links to the Surrealists, and a connoisseur of the arts. In the 1920s, the French Surrealists adopted hysteria as the model for their avant-garde art, a language of the unconscious and dreams opposed to science and the academies. In their 1928 manifesto, "Le cinquantenaire de l'hystérie," the poets Louis

Aragon and André Breton acclaimed hysteria as the "greatest poetic discovery of the nineteenth century."[49]

Beginning in 1964, Lacan presented a public seminar every Wednesday at the École normale supérieure. The feminist writer Catherine Clément attended regularly. As she recalls, "You had to get there quite early: an hour in advance was barely sufficient to get a seat. . . . The hall quickly filled to overflowing. Besides the psychoanalysts and the *normaliens*, curious at first and quickly conquered, there were actors and writers. With each new term new faces were added to the crowd." At these lectures, Lacan put forth his theories and case studies. "Having an audience," Clément notes, "gives a theatrical atmosphere to the event. Something of the spirit of Charcot is in the air: hysteria passes in review, offering bits and pieces of narrative as it struts upon the stage."[50]

At the École Freudienne, Lacan presided over a corps of devoted disciples and continued to see patients as well. He promoted his own arcane theories of hysteria, which had a tremendous influence on French intellectual life and especially on women analysts. He attempted to "hystericize" psychoanalysis, by which he meant restoring to it the playfulness, wildness, and mystery that had made it so exciting at the beginning of the century. On the theoretical level, Lacan gave hysteria pride of place in the psychoanalytic system. He believed hysteria, women, femininity, and gender were knotted together; the hysteric was most likely a woman struggling with her sexual identity.

But Lacan never created the alliance with hysterics that Charcot and Freud had achieved. He was the star of his lectures, unwilling to share the spotlight with hysterical performers. And although his ideas and his style certainly had a huge effect on French culture, and had their heyday in academe, Lacan's relentless difficulty and personal arrogance cut him off from the popular following others had won, and he might have gained.

Hysteria Today

Like it or not, we live in a psychoanalytic century. As Mark Micale and Roy Porter observe, "We turn to the psychosciences to run our private relationships, to raise our children, to try our criminals, to interpret our works of art, to improve our sex lives, to tell us why we are unhappy, depressed, anxious, or fatigued."[51] In the United States, the number of therapists has grown enormously during the past two decades. Although psychiatry, which demands a medical degree and special training, had a relatively modest increase between 1975 and 1990, the number of clinical psychologists almost tripled, and the number of clinical social workers and marriage and family counselors multiplied even more.[52]

But the expansion in mental health specialists has not produced consensus about hysteria. A century after Charcot and Freud, psychotherapists are still divided about what hysteria means and baffled by how it works. The twists and turns of psychoanalytic thought as it has attempted to come to terms with hysteria are interesting mainly to psychoanalysts, and probably even they find some of it tedious. Yet throughout the century, psychoanalysis has struggled to define hysterical syndromes, and despite attacks on Freud, the disorders he treated have continued to mutate. Though modified, the image of the doctor-guru is still strong in psychotherapy; every current hysterical syndrome has its own therapeutic advocates and promoters. As we shall see, the presence of these authority figures has been crucial to the growth of modern epidemic hysterias.

4

Politics, Patients, and Feminism

"Without the context of a political movement," writes Judith Lewis Herman, "it has
never been possible to advance the study of
psychological trauma."[1] For over a century, the political context for
hysteria has been feminism. Hysteria became a hot topic in medical circles during the 1880s and 1890s, when feminism, the New Woman, and
a crisis in gender were also hot topics in the United States and Europe.
Fin-de-siècle feminism coincided with the pseudoscientific discourses
of race degeneration: degenerationists believed that women's activ-
ism—particularly the fight to be admitted to universities and to enter
the professions—led to a decline in marriage and a falling birth rate.
Women, they argued, were cultivating their brains but neglecting their
biology. Conservatives saw feminism as the woman's form of degeneration; doctors viewed hysterical women as closet feminists who had to
be reprogrammed into traditional roles, and politicians attacked feminist activists as closet hysterics who needed treatment rather than
rights. The New Woman, one English journalist wrote, "ought to be
aware that her condition is morbid, or at least hysterical."[2]

In England at the turn of the century, hysteria, feminism, and
political speech merged in the popular mind. Women who spoke out
in public for women's rights were caricatured as "the shrieking sis-
terhood," a term coined by the English antifeminist novelist Eliza
Lynn Linton. In 1910 Arnold Ward warned that giving women the
vote would "incorporate that hysterical activity permanently into the

life of the nation."[3] In Austria, too, hysteria was blamed for women's pioneering efforts to become doctors. Fritz Wittels, a Viennese contemporary of Freud's, declared, "Hysteria is the basis for a woman's desire to study medicine, just as it is the basis of women's struggle for equal rights."[4]

New Women, intellectuals, and feminists like Olive Schreiner, Eleanor Marx, and Bertha Pappenheim were the most conspicuous of the women diagnosed as hysterics in England and Austria. American feminist intellectuals also consulted doctors: Morton Prince in Boston and Silas Weir Mitchell in Philadelphia specialized in treating women with artistic and literary aspirations who had mysterious symptoms of anxiety and depression. Although male physicians often suffered from hysteria, they blamed higher education and professional ambition for the epidemic of female nervous illness: "For me," Mitchell wrote in 1888, "the grave significance of sexual difference controls the whole question. . . . The woman's desire to be on a level of competition with man and to assume his duties is, I am sure, making mischief, for it is my belief that no length of generations of change in her education and modes of activity will ever really alter her characteristics. She is physiologically other than man."[5]

Doctors diagnosed the nervous complaints of female intellectuals and feminists as neurasthenia, a chronic fatigue syndrome first identified in the United States as "American nervousness" or N.E. (Nervous Exhaustion). Its origins can be traced at least to the 1870s, when the American neurologist George M. Beard argued that life in the fast lane for educated and professional men and women had precipitated mental and physical fatigue with organic causes beyond the diagnostic capacities of nineteenth-century medical science. Neurasthenia soon appeared in Europe, where it became the hysteria of the elite at the turn of the century.

Middle-class women might be called neurasthenics rather than hysterics, but however flattering the euphemism, female neurasthenia differed substantially from the male variety. Doctors defined its most significant causes as disturbances of reproduction and childbirth, emotional trauma, exhaustion, and intellectual strain. The Weir Mitchell rest cure, often prescribed for women intellectuals and artists in the United States and England, required the patient to spend six weeks or more in bed without any work, reading, or social life, and to gain large amounts of weight on a high-fat diet. Many women found the treatment itself maddening, and indeed Mitchell wanted the treatment to be more unpleasant than the symptoms so that patients would be eager to get out of bed.

Why were feminism and hysteria "two sides of the same coin or two ends of a continuum"? John Forrester and Lisa Appignanesi conclude that one reason was "the sexual conservatism of so much feminist activity."[6] They explain in *Freud's Women* that many late-nineteenth-century feminists also belonged to the temperance, hygiene, social purity, or eugenics movements, so that they attempted to embody ideals of asceticism and sexual morality. Living up to these ideals created unconscious conflicts that hysterical symptoms like paralysis or loss of voice might express.

American Hysterics

Changing sexual mores and attitudes toward appropriate roles for women affected both symptoms and treatment. In *The Psychiatric Persuasion: Knowledge, Gender and Power in Modern America* (1994), Princeton University historian Elizabeth Lunbeck studied Boston Psychopathic Hospital records from the early decades of this century. Although hysterical women made up less than 1 percent of the hospital's clientele, they were 25 percent of the case load of the hospital's only Freudian doctor, L. E. Emerson. His case studies reflect Freud's techniques of bullying women patients and pressuring them to come up with stories of sexual trauma. Emerson "urged women to sift through their memories . . . for the unpleasant sexual experiences that might help explain their ailments, and he expected women would find, then divulge, these memories quickly." When they did not, he blamed repression or ignored what they had to say. "Chews the rag," he complained about one patient. Although he theoretically understood the danger of influencing his patients, Emerson's records show "the mix of subtle suggestion and emotional incentives that in nearly every case yielded the information he sought." Because many of his patients were woefully ignorant about sexuality, and even about menstruation, Emerson felt that it was his duty to enlighten them; "to woman after woman he explained the facts of sex."

The women Emerson treated for hysteria were generally young, single, and white. About a third of them reported that they had been victims of sexual assault or incest. Another third reported sexual incidents with employers or boyfriends that they experienced as aggression, though these encounters fell within the bounds of "what men, and their culture, considered 'normal' heterosexuality." The last third were so terrified by adult female sexuality that they had withdrawn from courtship or heterosexual activity, despite longing for love and marriage. Lunbeck writes, "In a culture that nurtured male sexual aggressiveness and in which even heterosexual couplings that had been openly entered into were suffused with this aggression, it was sometimes difficult for women to draw a firm line between abuse on the one hand, and consensual sexual activity on the other." Psychiatrists responded unsympathetically to this dilemma of culture and gender because they themselves had inherited both a tradition of disdain for the hysterical woman and distrust of the sexual woman. Thus, Lunbeck concludes, "In psychiatrists' evolving discourse, the hypersexual and the hysteric served as emblematic representations of modern womanhood and its possibilities gone awry."[7]

Feminists Fight Back

How did women doctors and psychiatrists contend with epidemic hysteria? The feminist critique of the treatment of hysteria is at least a century old. Feminist activists in the antivivisection movement challenged Charcot's exploitation of hysterical women patients in the 1880s and 1890s. In 1888, a distinguished Russian woman scientist, Madame S. V. Kovalevskaia, gave a scathing account of her visit to the Salpêtrière: "Charcot is the master of this kingdom of neurosis," she noted. "To him all here relate with awe bordering on servility." She was embarrassed by his treatment of the women, especially charity cases, who had to put up with any humiliation: "He relates to them extremely unceremoniously; it never enters his head whether they feel things or not. He examines them, sounds their chests, exposes their ailments to the gaze of the students just as indifferently as if he were doing it to a mannequin, and right there in front of them gives his diagnosis and voices what are frequently very sad prognoses, not in the least worrying about what it means to them to hear their own sentences."[8]

Some women doctors came to study hysteria under Charcot and offered socially aware interpretations of its sources in women's restricted lives. Mademoiselle Georgette Déga argued that women's susceptibility to hysterical disorders was the result of their milieu and upbringing. Whatever women's social class, she explained in her doctor's thesis, all were "novices of hysteria," discouraged from making full use of their intellectual capacities, rewarded for developing their emotional side: "This female mode of reaction is called sensitivity and is encouraged and praised in women although it entails a disequilibrium of their psychic being."[9]

However, as a member of a minuscule group of women physicians, none of whom had an institutional base, Déga was unable to translate these insights into an effective and persuasive program. She certainly did not have the power and visibility of a Charcot. Thus instead of recommending a wider field of activity to women, she argued that girls should study mathematics and stop reading novels. In Martha Noel Evans's view, Déga revealed her own helplessness and ambivalence in this remedy. "Rather than turning the enormous strength she perceives in herself and in her patients outward in transforming action, she returns, in a self-punishing reversal, to a horrifying stiffening of women which tragically resembles the cataleptic state of the hysterics she set out to cure."[10]

What's much more surprising is that in the twentieth century, Freud's first female disciples—pioneering and influential women psychoanalysts such as Karen Horney, Melanie Klein, and Helene Deutsch—largely ignored hysteria. In a recent study, Nancy Chodorow suggests some explanations. Chodorow conducted interviews with forty-four women psychoanalysts trained in the 1920s through the mid-1940s, in the United States, Great Britain, and the Netherlands.[11] She found an absence of feminist awareness in these women analysts' lives that initially struck her as dismaying and incredible. They did not find it notable that many women became analysts in the early decades of the movement; they did not think the presence of women and/or mothers among the leading analysts had any significance for the field; they did not think of femininity as an aspect of their own professional histories; they had noticed very few gender differences in the way they were treated; they did not relate psychoanalytic theories of femininity and castration anxiety to their own careers or career motivations.

Eventually, Chodorow concluded that the women analysts' blindness to issues of gender represented concerns faced by their generation. During training, the profession gave no "theoretical prominence to gender or to gender-specific sexuality." Men and women clashed over the theory of femininity, but Chodorow insists that "most analysts of both sexes felt themselves actively engaged in other struggles that were more salient—in cultural and medical struggle, controversy and debate about Freud's theories of the unconscious and infantile sexuality. In these debates, they were certainly on Freud's side." On the whole, despite some prejudicial male attitudes, women analysts "clearly received substantial recognition." And their marital patterns allowed them to avoid some conflicts between maternity and professionalism. "Modally, they married in their early to mid-thirties, and had children in their mid-to-late thirties; even those who seem the most domestic members of psychoanalytic couples didn't marry until at least their late twenties. Thus their careers were already established by the time they were confronting the demands of motherhood."[12] In addition, having children was a functional solution to the Freudian dilemma; Lisa Appignanesi and John Forrester write, "For Freud there was no problem in a woman having a masculine identification once this was combined with motherhood."[13]

Becoming analysts represented for these women a radical break with their mothers' domestic lives, and moving into the public sphere satisfied their feminist impulses. "Participation in an exciting professional movement as equals and notions of socialist comradeship characterized their experience of work relations, women's natural roles as mothers and (equal but different) wives their experience of home roles. They assumed a division of labor in the home, assumed women's natural maternitality, assumed innate, and desirable, gender personality differences." Chodorow concluded that her own generation had been sensitized to feminist concerns in a way that had not existed before: "The pervasiveness of gender as a category to me simply did not resonate with their own life experiences, and I began to realize how much my perceptual and analytic categories had been shaped by my coming of age in the women's movement and my immersion in the recent literature of gender theory."[14]

The Herstory of Hysteria

Feminist academic interest in hysteria first emerged through the writing of women's history. Early in the women's liberation movement, reclaiming the hostile labels attached to rebellious or deviant women became a popular feminist strategy. Although "hysteria," like "witchcraft," had always been pejorative, it became a positive term for those trying to write the "her-story" of hysteria, a story that emphasized the cultural construction of women's hysterical symptoms, diagnosis, and treatment. Nineteenth-century hysterical women suffered from the lack of a public voice to articulate their economic and sexual oppression, and their symptoms—mutism, paralysis, self-starvation, spasmodic seizures—

seemed like bodily metaphors for the silence, immobility, denial of appetite, and hyperfemininity imposed on them by their societies.

Feminist historians focused especially on nineteenth-century America and England. What the cultural historian Ann Douglas called the "fashionable diseases" of nineteenth-century women were Victorian versions of hysterical complaint. In 1973, Douglas kicked off a lively debate about male doctors' complicity in creating and maintaining the disorders. Did these doctors despise their patients? Did they invent punitive treatments to express their own hostilities toward female discontent?

From a more sociological perspective, feminists have seen hysteria as the product of nineteenth-century conflicts over sex roles and female sexuality. According to historian Carroll Smith-Rosenberg, many American women escaped the realities of adult life by regressing to hysterical illness. In her view the clash between women's sheltered upbringing and their real domestic responsibilities "may have made the petulant infantilism and narcissistic self-assertion of the hysteric a necessary social alternative to women who felt unfairly deprived of their promised social role and who had few strengths with which to adapt to a more trying one."[15] Medical sociologists today argue that women are more likely to seek medical and therapeutic help, and thus to predominate in statistical studies. On the other hand, Mark Pendergrast suggests that women may actually be conduits for the hysteria of a culture; women, he writes, have long been socially encouraged to "act out the 'symptom pool' of the era and accept an inappropriate diagnosis."[16]

Reviewing feminist scholarship of the 1970s, medical historian Nancy Tomes finds an impasse over a fundamental contradiction:

> In these early works, feminist historians wrestled long and hard with the implications of interpreting women's nervous conditions as modes of protest against their limited gender roles. The notion of mental illness as a form of "protofeminism" had an obvious appeal. The well-known cases of talented women . . . who had nervous breakdowns and recovered only by forging unconventional lives for themselves seemed to suggest that feminism and madness were two sides of the same coin.

But the escape to madness was a costly one:

> The difficulties of reconciling these two interpretations of female madness remained a fundamental ambiguity in feminist portrayals of nineteenth-century psychiatry and its treatment of women.[17]

understand, any opinion that was contrary to their own."[45] Victor Lewis-Smith, the dreadlocked television critic for the *Evening Standard*, denounced the program as a travesty of investigative journalism: "There was no desire to seek the truth, merely to belittle and indoctrinate in an ill-considered, inconsiderate, manipulative, and unscrupulous manner."[46] Lewis-Smith was so outraged that he protested to the Broadcasting Complaints Commission.

Dr. Anne McIntyre, the medical adviser for the ME Association, responded that "the current battle going on is akin to the hostility people with multiple sclerosis experienced 40 or 50 years ago when they were described as hysterical because their symptoms came and went. No one would dare to describe their illness as imaginary now." But Stuttaford sees her assumption that psychologically-caused illness is "imaginary" as part of the problem. The audience was hostile, he said, "because there are people who have not yet learned to regard psychiatric disease as a proper illness. They are still seeing it as a moral weakness."[47] Spurning the idea that they can be helped by psychotherapy and antidepressants, chronic fatigue patients may go on for years, becoming more and more invested in the fruitless quest for a medical breakthrough. At some point, although the initial causes of the symptoms may have disappeared, the syndrome itself becomes a self-perpetuating reality.

Caught in a cultural impasse over the meaning of their symptoms, many sufferers are understandably grateful to find a Reverend Bill. Faith healing is a cheap price to pay for being rescued from a disorder that has baffled medical opinion. Although sources of the fatigue may have disappeared, patients cannot easily discard their symptoms without some kind of face-saving intervention.

Chronic Fatigue: The Doctors

Doctors and other health workers have always been peculiarly susceptible to neurasthenia and other chronic fatigue syndromes. In both England and the United States, doctors who have themselves been sufferers are advisers to the patient associations. Ten percent of George Beard's neurasthenic patients in the 1880s were doctors, and both Beard and S. Weir Mitchell had overcome the disorder. In the 1980s, Dr. Melvyn Ramsay, late president of the British Myalgic Encephalomyelitis Association asserted that "the incidence of ME among doctors is out of all proportion to their numbers in the general population."

Paul Cheney specifies personal experience as the difference between the physician who "believes" in CFS as an organic illness and those who see it as a psychological syndrome. "The only people who really believe in this disease are the few clinicians who have seen enough patients to have seen the pattern, and isolated clinicians who either have the disease themselves or who have someone close to them who has it," he told Johnson. "Once you believe this disease is real, your whole attitude changes. If you get a negative result or an ambiguous finding, you say, 'Well, it's a negative result or an ambiguous finding,' and you keep going, because you know the disease is real." Clearly, what is at stake is an unwillingness to accept a psychological disorder as "real," and a view of the disorders of psychiatry as unreal forms of malingering or deceit.

Nonetheless, the majority of doctors and researchers maintain that CFS is a psychological syndrome, *and* that its symptoms and effects are real. In the mid-1980s, Stephen E. Straus had encouraged researchers to pursue the connection to Epstein-Barr virus and other immune dysfunctions, but by 1988 he concluded that "it is impossible to completely dispel the notion that the chronic fatigue syndrome represents a psychoneurotic condition." In a 1995 address at the American College of Rheumatology, Straus reiterated his view that CFS was "not a [single] disease entity but a mixed bag of entities." He spoke of the CDC's inability to replicate experiments that showed the presence of retroviruses or brain damage. Straus's caveats have drawn angry rebuttals from Hillary Johnson, who accuses him of bias, "hostility towards his study subjects, a majority of whom were women," and "propaganda" about the patients' psychiatric condition.[48]

A state-of-the-art analysis of chronic fatigue syndrome emerged from a 1992 symposium at the Ciba Foundation in London, attended by an international group of outstanding physicians, psychiatrists, medical historians, anthropologists, virologists, and biologists. The conference set out to devise a coping plan for the treatment of chronic fatigue, a cognitive therapy that would direct itself to behaviors rather than causes. Professor Arthur Kleinman, from the departments of anthropology and social medicine at Harvard, set the stage from the patient's perspective: "Imagine being a chronic fatigue patient. . . . We go to see a doctor and are sent on to a psychiatrist. All of a sudden, the fundamental illness experience we have is no longer the grounds of our talk; we are being asked about our families, our intimate personal life, our fears, our worries. We sense a distortion or incongruity about where our experience is located: it's in the *fatigue*. And the psychiatrist, just by his or her position, challenges and even alienates us, and makes us feel that our experience, our primary grounding in our bodies, is unreal, imaginary."

Kleinman strongly believes that CFS should be treated by a physician, not by a psychiatrist, to maintain the patient's self-respect. "One can affirm the illness experience," he concludes, "without affirming the attribution for it; in other words, we can work within a 'somatic' language and do all the interventions that we heard earlier had been done from the psychosocial side, but in such a way as to spare patients the . . . delegitimization of their experience."[49]

David Mechanic, a distinguished sociologist of medicine at Rutgers University, adds: "In order to convince people who have a psychological and even monetary stake in believing in CFS as a viral condition, one has to provide a plausible alternative theory which they find credible. Much as my inclination is to believe that CFS is influenced by psychological needs, I am not convinced that there isn't an important viral trigger or a viral perpetuating factor. . . . I see no reason why the public should give up that belief, when you don't have anything particularly good to offer in return."[50]

But these kindly, tolerant, and temporizing views do not address the ways that psychogenic epidemics escalate. Doctors may protect the self-esteem of their patients in the short run by prescribing placebos like vitamins and avoiding public statements about the history of effort syndromes. But in the long run, such acquiescence only creates more hysteries. Modern psychological epidemics feed endlessly on new disease theories, such as immunology. Studies published in the *British Medical Journal* have shown that patients who believed their conditions were viral or infectious, and who became inactive, were least likely to have recovered after three years. Furthermore, in Wessely's view, "Such uncritical diagnoses may reinforce maladaptive behavior, and may create more severe and persistent morbidity than the initial illness."[51]

In *Osler's Web*, Johnson laments that "well into the 1990s, the story of the American epidemic and the people whose lives it destroyed continued to play out in a kind of half-light, unseen and unfelt in most regions of the culture . . . as a group [sufferers] inhabited a domain utterly removed from the mainstream."[52] But despite her claims of the twilight of CFS, it has not faded from the headlines and is unlikely to disappear anytime soon. Studies of CFS regularly identify and alert new victims. In a typically uncritical London *Times* article, a journalist reports that "at least 24,000 children in Britain" are suffering from ME, and that this may be "only the tip of the iceberg."

The figures come from a study by Elizabeth Dowsett, a microbiologist who "firmly believes" that ME is caused by enteroviral infections, and Jane Colby, a schoolteacher who suffers from the syndrome. Although a pediatrician specializing in ME is quoted as saying the "wide range and varying severity of symptoms can make diagnosis difficult," Dowsett nonetheless recommends "total rest" for a child with any of the symptoms: "Forcing a child to participate in lessons, PE, and 'normal' day-to-day activities will only make things worse." In her blanket warnings to parents, one can easily see an invitation to create invalidism in children, a Munchhausen-by-proxy syndrome. Dowsett says, "If the child has a rapid pulse or heartbeat, overexertion can be very dangerous. . . . So can exercising muscles before they're fully recovered, which, in extreme cases, can lead to paralysis. Also the stress of leading a normal life and keeping up with their peers can exacerbate the condition."[53] With scare literature like this, we can be sure that the anxious parents of many more children will soon be talking to doctors about ME.

Johnson herself points to the next adult phase of expansion for CFS: Gulf War syndrome. Toward the end of her book, in 1994 the story moves to New Jersey, where Dr. Benjamin Natalson has a $2.5 million grant from the NIH to study the relationship between chronic fatigue syndrome and Gulf War syndrome. "We think there has been a mini-epidemic of CFS among Gulf War veterans," Natalson says.[54] The epidemic stage is set for act two.

9

Gulf War Syndrome

"We've kicked Vietnam syndrome!" exulted President Bush in 1991, referring to American malaise after the disaster of Vietnam. But although most of its symptoms emerged later, the Persian Gulf conflict clearly marked the beginning of an unexplained illness that has been named Gulf War syndrome. In the summer of 1991, Brian Martin returned from Iraq to his family in Niles, Michigan. He was happy to be home but had a mysterious rash that wouldn't go away. During the next months other symptoms followed—memory lapses, mood swings, and finally debilitating fatigue. He can't work and gets some disability pay from the VA. But even worse symptoms have afflicted Brian's family. His son Deven, conceived shortly after Brian's return, was born with acute respiratory problems and an umbilical cord five feet long. His twenty-five-year-old wife, Kim, has suffered from seemingly unrelated and unconfirmed complaints—rashes, headaches, breast lumps, ovarian cysts, a thinning skull, and unexplained cervical infections. Now the Martins no longer have sex; after intercourse, Kim experiences cramps and a burning sensation: when her husband's semen touches her skin, she told *Redbook*, it feels "like it was on fire."[1] Doctors have been unable to find organic causes for any of the Martins' problems.

In Barrington, Illinois, the Albuck family is also suffering. Gulf War veteran Troy has fatigue, muscle soreness, swollen joints, headaches, diarrhea, and bleeding gums. His wife, Kelli, has hearing problems, migraines, and attacks of pelvic inflammatory disease. She reports that her husband's semen is a toxic substance that "causes sores—blisters which actually open and bleed." Worst of all, their son Alex was born prematurely in 1993 with a rare blood infection and now has cerebral palsy. When he was born, he had a rash that looked like the ones Troy and Kelli have had. Journalist David France declares that "doctors have been unable to explain their cause, give a diagnosis, or prescribe a remedy."[2]

In Yorkshire, England, Robert Lake's marriage has broken up since he returned from the Persian Gulf, plagued by headaches, vomiting, and diarrhea. Lake had become an army apprentice at sixteen and trained in Cyprus and Germany, where he moved at nineteen. Serving as a radar technician in the Gulf, he was shocked and frightened. On return, he began to have violent mood swings and nightmares of running away from an enemy; he made two suicide attempts and spent two months in psychiatric hospitals, where he was treated for PTSD. He continued to have angry outbursts, his German wife left him, and the army discharged him in 1993. Lake has lost about seventy pounds and has been diagnosed with anorexia nervosa. But he believes that his symptoms come from anthrax inoculations and antinerve gas tablets he took in the Gulf. "I am angry and disappointed," he told *The Guardian*, "that the MOD [Ministry of Defence] are so pig ignorant and uncaring."[3]

The Martins, the Albucks, and Robert Lake are among the thousands of American and British victims of what is called Gulf War syndrome (GWS), Saudi flu, or desert fever. Of the 697,000 U.S. troops who served in the Gulf, 60,000 have reported ailments from memory loss to cancer. The numbers in England are much smaller: 567 veterans, out of 45,000 British personnel, are seeking compensation or disability payments. Veterans' complaints include chronic fatigue, diarrhea, aches and pains, headaches, hair loss, bleeding gums, irritability, insomnia, muscle spasms, and night sweats. Two veterans in Mississippi have claimed to be shrinking.[4] Among physicians, politicians, journalists, and veterans who believe that Gulf War syndrome is a new and unique illness, ideas about its cause vary. Many believe that it is contagious and can be passed through sex, sweat, or the air.

Like CFS patients, Gulf War veterans have organized self-help networks. In 1994 David France reported in *Redbook* that "many vets rely on an informal word-of-mouth network to track the illness, tally developments, or find solace."[5] Veterans and their families who live on military bases trade stories, and electronic networks of Gulf War vets are humming; the Internet has hugely expanded opportunities to communicate. Most veterans and their families react angrily to the idea that they are suffering from post-traumatic stress disorder. Willie Hicks, a black veteran from Alabama, told *Esquire* journalist Gregory Jaynes, "Shit, I don't sleep more than two, three hours a day. Anxiety. . . . Couldn't get along with nobody. . . . Couldn't even get out the house. . . . Post-traumatic stress, my black ass."[6] Carole Hill, an English nurse who began to feel tired six months after her husband returned to Cheshire from the Gulf, insists: "This can't be psychological. I've spoken to too many veterans whose families are suffering similar symptoms."[7]

GWS patients in England and the U.S. are convinced that the cause of their medical problems lies in their exposure to chemicals and drugs in the Gulf, and that their governments are conspiring to deprive them of health benefits and disability pay. Hicks says angrily, "Some of us bleed from the penis. Bleed all over the sheets. Government won't even pay for the sheets."[8] "We believe there's a cover-up," British-born Texan Vic Silvester tells *The Guardian*[9]. "I was a volunteer, so I have to take whatever I get," one American veteran says. "But my boy and my wife? They did not volunteer, they did not take my oath. They've been drafted against their will and they've got wounds from battle."[10] A group of sick wives in Texas has started its own secret research initiative—"secret," according to one of them, "because they fear the military might try to block their study for reasons she can only guess at."[11]

In fact, American government reactions to Gulf War syndrome have been concerned and sympathetic. No elected politician wants to risk his constituents' anger. The Clinton administration, mindful of alienation over Vietnam and the Agent Orange fiasco, has moved very carefully. President Clinton authorized a scientific advisory panel to investigate the symptoms. Hillary Rodham Clinton has come out as a "friend of Gulf War syndrome sufferers." At the opening session of the Presidential Committee meeting, she said, "Just as we relied on our troops when they were sent to war, we must assure them that they can rely on us now."[12] Politicians agree that Persian Gulf veterans deserve respect, attention, and full support, and no decent citizen could object to the research efforts and investigations funded by the government. Since 1994, the government has authorized disability payments for veterans with GWS.

The respectful and cautious responses of the U.S. government, however, have reinforced the suspicion that Gulf War syndrome is a unique disease and fed anxieties and conspiracy rumors about it. Dissenting views have been silenced; when Dr. Edward Young, chief of staff at the Houston VA Medical Center, announced, "There's been mass hallucinations. There's been mass post-traumatic stress disorder" and attributed some of the epidemic to frustration and anger, he was suspended by his boss, Jesse Brown, secretary of the Department of Veterans' Affairs.[13] But more skeptical responses of the British Defence Ministry have not quelled protests from MPs or veterans either.

The extraordinary conditions of the Gulf War—and Iraq's admission that they had biological weapons they didn't use—have added to suspicions that GWS is caused by a toxic agent. These concerns and questions reappeared when the Pentagon announced in June 1996 that a weapons storage area exploded by American troops contained toxic gases. But there is no clinical evidence that GWS soldiers were exposed to the blast nor that the minute traces of sarin and mustard gas could have caused the enormous variety of symptoms being reported by thousands of veterans five years later. In a "Sixty Minutes" special on August 25, 1996, a group of soldiers from the 37th Engineers Batallion who participated in blowing up an Iraqi arsenal near Kamisayah in March 1991 described their fears at the time of the demolition, and a variety of symptoms since. But CBS did not interview any doctors, specialists in the effects of nerve gas, or Pentagon officials who could support the claim that this chemical exposure could lead to fatigue, gastrointestinal symptoms, and other problems. What has seemed likely all along is that no one incident, toxin, virus, or disease entity is responsible for all the complaints that have been collected under the heading of Gulf War syndrome.[14]

Meanwhile doctors are pursuing many other explanations. Dr. Edward Hyman of New Orleans, who believes the syndrome is an arterial infection passed through the air like tuberculosis, has been voted $1.2 million by Congress for research.[15] Ross Perot is among those funding a Mayo Clinic project. Dr. Boaz Milner in Allen Park, Michigan, has treated more than three hundred GWS patients. He has suggested at least five possible causes for Gulf War syndrome: radiation poisoning, effects of experimental medicines, environmental contaminants, chemical compounds, and Iraq's biological arsenal. Dr. Eula Bingham, a professor of environmental health at the University of Cincinnati, suspects leishmaniasis, a parasitic infection caused by sand fly bites; but the Armed Forces Epidemiological Board says no. Researchers at Duke have found that the experimental nerve gas pill pyrodostigmine bromide, used in combination with pesticides, caused neurological problems in chickens. When Dr. Stephen C.

Joseph, assistant secretary of defense for health affairs, responded that pyrodostigmine stays in the human body for only a few hours, the next suggestion was multiple chemical sensitivity. One entomologist reported that an insect repellent used by 40 percent of the soldiers in the Gulf becomes more toxic when mixed with pyrodostigmine.[16] Among the latest stories is that aspartame, an artificial sweetener used in Nutrasweet, is linked to GWS. Now that Hillary Johnson and others are pointing out correspondences with chronic fatigue syndrome, researchers are investigating retroviruses.

Yet government investigations have produced no evidence of an organic syndrome. Dr. Francis Murphy, acting director of the office of environmental medicine and public health at the VA says, "We have found nothing in our investigations that we consider transmissible. We've found no clear-cut evidence that this is being transmitted either casually or sexually."[17] A defense department study of more than a thousand ailing veterans indicated that 60 percent had organic ailments with known causes, which were not disproportionate to their random occurrence in the population. Another 25 percent had psychological disturbances, including depression and post-traumatic stress disorder. About 15 percent had unexplained ailments, including headache, memory loss, fatigue, sleep problems, and intestinal and respiratory complaints.[18] In January 1995, a panel affiliated with the National Academy of Sciences recommended a fuller and more coordinated study of the problem.[19] By April 1996, the results were announced: conducted at a cost of $80 million, the survey of 18,924 veterans found "no single cause or mystery ailment to support suspicions about the existence of a gulf war syndrome."[20]

In England, results were similar. "I have seen or heard nothing that makes me believe there is a specific syndrome directly attributable to the gulf war," says surgeon-general Tony Revell. A Ministry of Defence study indicated that about 52 percent of those surveyed had minor ailments like asthma. Fourteen percent had more serious disorders, including leukemia and kidney disease. Solicitor Hilary Meredith, whose law firm represents 567 veterans, say nine have died from cancer. Twenty-two percent had post-traumatic stress disorder, and 14 percent had other psychological symptoms, including depression and anxiety.[21] In July 1995, the Royal College of Physicians gave its official backing for further investigations, although a preliminary study had concluded that "there was no single cause for the variety of illnesses suffered by the servicemen and women who have been examined."[22]

Gulf War Syndrome and Shell Shock

Many of these symptoms sound like war neurosis, shell shock, or post-traumatic stress disorder. Despite the rapidity with which PTSD has entered the language, most people do not understand what it means or know about its long history: from the Civil War on, battle fatigue, shell shock, combat neurosis, or PTSD has been observed, studied, and documented, not only in American medicine and psychiatry but around the world.

Since the Gulf War, however, journalists, doctors, government officials, and psychologists have been surprisingly silent about PTSD. Instead, the media have exacerbated fears of Gulf War symptoms. By the summer of 1995, more than two hundred newspaper stories about Gulf War syndrome had appeared in England.[23] Even *Doonesbury* picked up on the controversy, with B.D. complaining to Boopsie about his symptoms and denying that they could be caused by stress: "It doesn't explain why this thing is showing up in family members too! I'm terrified I might end up passing it on to you!"

In the United States, both conservative and liberal journalists have long promoted the idea that Gulf War syndrome is a contagious disease being covered up by the government. In *Redbook* David France asks why the VA has not authorized semen tests on veterans. In the feminist *Women's Review of Books*, Laura Flanders writes, "Today many women who served in the Gulf are still in combat, only this time their fight is with the Department of Defense and the Veterans Administration.... After months of struggle and increasing sickness, the tears are now of rage."[24] Flanders has also written about GWS for *The Nation*, where she declares that "fears are growing about just how contagious Gulf War Syndrome may be. Outgoing Senator Donald Riegel conducted a study of 1,200 sick male veterans last year and found that 78 percent of their wives had been affected.... Penny Larrissey, a veteran's wife who told me last year that during intercourse her husband's semen burns, has been in touch with military wives around the country who report not just discomfort but terrible vaginal infections, cysts, blisters and even bleeding sores. Most military family members remain outside the national test samples. And some are invisible altogether. Thanks to the Pentagon's devotion to discrimination, gay men and lesbians whose partners are sick are too scared to ask for help and too intimidated to tell."[25]

This kind of journalism makes classic hystory: scare headlines, vague statistics, uncritical descriptions of "studies" and "reports," and the extension of anxieties to gays in the military. Perceptions are reported as facts; undifferentiated and unsubstantiated responses taken seriously as medical evidence. Senator Riegel's staff, for example, surveyed six hundred veterans, 77 percent of whom *said* that their spouses had some symptoms. On the page opposite Flanders's story, an ad claims, "The most skeptical people in America subscribe to *The Nation.*" One has to wonder why.

Some of the most alarmist, upsetting, and irresponsible journalism has been about birth defects related to GWS. Immediately after the war, there were persistent rumors of birth defects among the families of returning veterans. Laura Flanders notes dramatically that "freakish births are being reported around the country and even internationally."[26] In November 1995, *Life* magazine published a special issue entitled "The Tiny Victims of Desert Storm: Has Our Country Abandoned Them?" On the cover was a color picture of Gulf War veteran Sgt. Paul Hanson and his three-year-old-son Jayce, born with hands and feet attached to stumps. In the story, heart-rending photos of Jayce, "the unofficial poster boy of the Gulf War babies," accompany text full of dire warning and no firm medical or statistical evidence. "During the past year," the story says, "*Life* has conducted its own inquiry into the plight of these children. We sought to learn whether U.S. policies put them at risk, and whether the nation ought to be doing more for them and their families."

The story describes the anguish of seven families whose children have birth defects, from spinal bifida to mitral heart valve disorder. But reporters Jimmie Briggs and Kenneth Miller do not provide numbers of complaints or controls, although they sneer at "Pentagon bureaucrats" who claim that "at least 3 percent of American babies are born with abnormalities." One activist group, the Association of Birth Defect Children, has gathered data on ailing babies born to 163 of the 970,000 who served in the Gulf War. According to *Life,* "No one . . . knows how many babies have been born to Gulf vets," and "many still question whether Defense Department scientists are really seeking the hard answers,"[27] despite more than thirty studies of Gulf vets by 1995.

Esquire reported in 1994 that "of fifty-five children born to four Guard Units in Mississippi thirty-seven are not normal."[28] According to the Mississippi Department of Public Health, however, two babies in these units were born with severe defects and three with minor defects. The VA maintained in May 1994 that the percentage of birth defects in the Mississippi units fell within the normal range—a conclusion that "enraged" one mother, who argued that birth defect statistics were not the point: "Our babies are sick all the time. Why didn't they study our children's immune systems?" Dr. Alan Penman, director of a study by the Centers for Disease Control and Prevention, responded: "We don't believe that there's an excessively high rate of common illnesses in this group."[29]

Angry parents like Ammie West, whose daughter Reed was born with a chronic respiratory infection, have condemned the Mississippi study, like other government statistics and responses that offer facts and reassurance, as part of a cover-up. A Pentagon survey of the army's six largest military installations showed that the rate of spontaneous abortion or miscarriage among veterans' wives was about half the rate of society as a whole. But, says David France, "This result has been denounced by vets as a partial finding at best."[30] Parents are understandably anxious and grief-stricken, but we have to question the usefulness of scare stories.

Journalists could be more helpful by reminding readers of the atmosphere leading up to the Gulf War and the many forces that contributed to stress and disorientation for participants. In a report on 10,020 Gulf War participants issued in August 1995, the defense department announced, "Physical and psychological stressors were major characteristics of the Persian Gulf. The effect of both acute and chronic stress is a major etiologic consideration when evaluating Persian Gulf veterans. U.S. troops entered a bleak, physically demanding desert environment, where they were crowded into warehouses, storage buildings, and tents with little personal privacy and few amenities. No one knew that coalition forces eventually would win a quick war with relatively few battle casualties. Consequently, most troops did not fight a 'four day war' but spent months isolated in the desert, under constant stress, concerned about their survival and their family's well-being at home, and uncertain about when they would return home."[31]

In an article for the London *Times*, Dr. Simon Wessely reminds us just how stressful service in the Persian Gulf was. Troops were afraid that Iraq might use devastating chemical and biological weapons, and "to be ever alert for a silent attack by nerve gas or invisible deadly microbes must have taken a constant toll. . . . The situation was made worse by the cumbersome protection suits, ill-adapted for the desert heat, that had to be worn as a consequence."[32]

Testimony from Gulf War veterans with GWS confirms these descriptions. Seventeen percent of Gulf War forces came from National Guard reserve units who had never expected to be on active duty, especially under such ominous conditions. They had heard about the ruthlessness of Saddam Hussein and his unbeatable "elite Republican Guard." That Saddam's troops proved to be ill-equipped and outnumbered did not undo the months of fearful anticipation. Iraqi Scud attacks on civilian populations intensified fears of a bestial enemy, while propaganda about biological and chemical warfare made every new experience potentially threatening. Soldiers also had to deal with frightening gossip about the preventive medications offered to them.

One Hingham, Massachusetts, soldier, Larry McGinnis, took eight of the anti–nerve gas pills—more than the recommended dose—and vomited for several hours. "Here we were," he told a reporter, "driving into Iraq with the 82nd Airborne and me puking over the side into the sand. . . . I thought I was going to die."[33] McGinnis had reason to fear death. In his testimony to the House Subcommittee of the Committee on Veterans' Affairs, he recalled crossing the DMI "with the thought of the body bags and coffins that were being delivered. . . . But the one thought that kept coming back was Gas Chemical Warfare."[34]

Women too had profoundly disturbing combat experiences. Sergeant Carol Picou, an army medical officer, drove a hospital truck into Iraq, where she saw charred and smoldering bodies of animals and humans beside the highway. Although Picou had seen burned bodies before, she was frightened: "These bodies were different. They weren't normal." For two weeks Picou and her unit lived near the battlefield, treating injured soldiers and Iraqi civilians from Basra. After she returned from the Gulf, Picou began to suffer from muscle pain, bladder problems, and memory loss. She is convinced that her symptoms were caused not by horror, anxiety, and disgust but by the drug pyrodostigmine.[35]

Gulf War syndrome is shaping up to be a tragic standoff of men and women suffering from the all-too-real aftereffects of war, doctors unable to combat the force of rumor and panic, and a government that feels the need to be supportive of veterans. As Representative Joseph Kennedy told the House Subcommittee, "They come back, were told when they begin to complain of various illnesses that these can be explained through PTSD or through stress. It's one thing for us to hear that. It's another thing, if you've got all these sicknesses . . . and you are being told by a doctor that you go in to see at the VA that, listen, there is nothing really wrong with you—all it is, you know, you've got some psychological problem that is getting in your way—which must be an enormous burden for these individuals to carry around. . . . Now if in the end the conclusion is that these are illnesses that are explained only through PTSD, that might be the conclusion but it seems to me that we are a long way from drawing that conclusion at the moment."[36]

That was in the fall of 1992. Years have gone by, but each time the government eliminates a chemical or bacterial cause, suspicion, resistance, and bitterness grows. As Paul Cotton commented in a 1994 report in the *Journal of the American Medical Association*, the Pentagon's effort to reassure Persian Gulf veterans seems to have "created a candy store for conspiracy buffs." Among the persistent rumors surrounding GWS are stories of 2,000 concealed deaths among Gulf veterans, mass burials of contaminated Iraqi bodies, the release of a Russian chemical called Novachok, mysterious deaths of camels and goats in the desert, exposure to depleted uranium, the use of soldiers as guinea pigs for unauthorized drugs or vaccines, and widespread burning of soldiers' medical records.[37] Meanwhile, thousands of men and women who could be helped by psychotherapy are instead encouraged to pursue endless tests and medical exams; they tend not to see psychotherapists even when their stories make clear that anxiety, fear, and anger are among their symptoms.

Studies have shown that "very substantial proportions of Vietnam veterans with readjustment problems" have never sought help from mental health specialists. Ignorance of therapy, fear of stigma, ideas about masculine self-sufficiency, and lack of information were the main reasons veterans did not seek help. "By far the most frequently reported reason . . . was the hope or belief that the individual could solve the problem on his own. . . . Other major reasons . . . were feeling as though treatment would not help, not knowing where to get help, distrust of mental health professionals, the respondent's fear of what he might learn from consulting a mental health professional, and the time and cost involved in seeking treatment."[38] Education could have changed the way veterans perceived themselves and allowed them to seek care without feeling diminished as men. We do not want the same ignorance and misinformation to persist for Gulf War veterans.

We owe our war veterans a serious debt, but continuing to deny the validity of war neurosis is not the way to pay it. The suffering of Gulf War syndrome *is* real by any measure, and the symptoms caused by war

12

Satanic Ritual Abuse

In 1986, therapists gathered in Chicago at the International Conference on Multiple Personality/Dissociation noticed a surprising development: about 25 percent of their MPD patients were describing memories of torture and abuse in secret satanic cults. Rather than feeling disturbed by these stories and the lack of evidence to support them, large numbers of therapists incorporated satanic ritual abuse (SRA) into their theoretical and psychological repertoire. The 1986 conference had one paper on satanic ritual abuse; a year later, there were eleven. By 1989, George Ganaway, director of the Center for Dissociative Studies at the University of Georgia, disclosed that almost half the patients in his clinic and elsewhere were "reporting vividly detailed memories of cannibalistic revels and extensive experiences such as being used by cults during adolescence as serial baby breeders for ritual sacrifices." Therapists kept up with patients by organizing seminars and publishing articles and books to circulate information and educate other mental health professionals about the problem. In *Out of Darkness: Exploring Satanism and Ritual Abuse* (1992), editors David Sakheim and Susan E. Devine described their field as "in its infancy."[1] But many psychiatrists in the field were skeptical, and the multiple movement is still divided over the truth of satanic ritual abuse.

The media soon got involved. "All over the country," wrote reporter Leslie Bennetts in 1993, "what seems to be an astonishing number of women are coming forward with similar tales of satanic cults and ritual abuse. The reports are being made by all kinds of women—

different socioeconomic backgrounds, different ethnicities, different religions, even different races.... Over and over again, women told me about being forced to kill and eat babies at satanic ceremonies, about seeing children dismembered and boiled and burned, about being drugged, tortured with cattle prods, branded with branding irons, raped with crucifixes and animal carcasses. They told me about being buried in coffins with live snakes and dead bodies, about being tied to crosses and hung upside down for days, about being photographed for child pornographers and caged by satanic child-prostitution rings that farmed out their tiny victims for further abuse."[2]

After the 1983 McMartin preschool case in California—finally dismissed seven years and $15 million later for lack of evidence—other women charged that their children had been ritually abused in day care centers or nursery schools. Then came sensational investigations by well-meaning but overzealous police, doctors, and social workers who performed rectal and genital examinations on the children, invited them to demonstrate what had happened with anatomically correct dolls, and asked leading questions. The first edition of *The Courage to Heal*, in 1988, quoted San Francisco policewoman Sandi Gallant:"People say children invent these stories after watching TV, but before there was any media coverage of these cases, the allegations these kids made were extremely consistent with the allegations other kids were making in other parts of the country.... Children don't make up stories like these."[3]

Satanic ritual abuse stories also caught on in Britain. In Rochdale, near Manchester, twenty children were taken out of their homes in 1990 by social workers after a six-year-old boy told teachers that he had seen babies murdered, children drugged and caged, and people digging up graves. The claims were dismissed after a ten-week hearing in the High Court. In the remote Orkney Islands in 1991, nine children were removed from their homes after a villager reported peculiar practices by families that included Jews and Quakers. Children told investigators about participating in satanic rites with people dressed as Ninja Turtles. After an inquiry that cost six million pounds, charges against the adults were dismissed and social workers were criticized for their suggestive questions. In some cases, the pressures of evangelical Christians, along with the influence of horror films, evidently supplied the imagery and plot for imaginary narratives.[4]

From accusations of devil worshipers molesting children in day care centers, to agitation over rumors about the kidnaping and sacrifice of a blond, blue-eyed virgin, to talk of animal mutilation and ritual sexual abuse, the United States was rocked with stories of satanism and witchcraft in the late 1980s. Exacerbated by sensational TV programs and by fundamentalist "experts" on satanism, the hysteria moved from small town to small town, leaving frightened children and parents in its wake. Two kinds of stories combined in the epidemic: charges by children, and recovered memories of adults who had remembered nothing prior to therapy.

As witch-hunters' accusations become wilder and wilder, as courts reject lawsuit after lawsuit for lack of evidence, many therapists have become uneasy. Years of lawsuits and intensive investigations have unearthed no proof that these satanic cults even exist. Kenneth V. Lanning, special agent at the FBI Behavioral Science Unit in Quantico, Virginia, has studied over 300 SRA allegations since 1983, and has found no evidence to corroborate them. In 1994, the British government released a report based on a three-year inquiry into eighty-four cases of alleged SRA. The study—chaired by Dr. Jean La Fontaine, author of a respected book on child abuse and professor emeritus of social anthropology at the London School of Economics—found no evidence to support any of the charges. "It's a national scandal," says American psychiatric social worker Jan Larsen. "With all the satanic ritual-abuse cases, there's not a shred of evidence. I don't think it exists. I think it's hysterical contamination, but it's making people sick, making money, and hurting families."[5] Therapist George Ganaway warns, "Unless scientifically documented proof is forthcoming, patients and therapists who validate and publicly defend the unsubstantiated veracity of these reports may find themselves developing into a cult of their own, validating each others' beliefs while ignoring (and being ignored by) the scientific and psychotherapeutic community at large."[6]

What is the hystory of satanic ritual abuse? According to John Briere's widely used textbook *Therapy for Adults Molested as Children* (1989), patients describe "black magic or satanic rites, where the child victim is part of a ceremony involving desecration and sexual debasement. Examples of such activities include the child being forced to publicly masturbate with a crucifix; ceremonial gang rape by all (or a privileged few) of the male members of the cult; sexual contact with or dismemberment of a family pet; demands that the child drink blood or urine or eat vile substances; and ritualistic ceremonies where the child is stripped of clothing, tied to a crucifix or platform, sexually molested, and led to believe that she is about to be sacrificed."[7] Satanic cult stories also may refer to brainwashing, programming, and hypnotic or post-hypnotic suggestion.

With their thematic emphasis on incest, infanticide, forced breeding, cannibalism, and conspiracy, these narratives touch on the deepest and most frightening taboos and fantasies of our culture.[8] Alleged victims of satanic cults describe conspiracies by huge, intergenerational, secretive criminal organizations that maintain total control over their members and victims; leaders avoid detection by living in disguise as normal members of the community. Fears of punishment and revenge by the cult for betraying its secrets become so vivid in clinical settings that hospital workers themselves begin to develop hypervigilant panics. In *Shattered Selves*, University of Maryland professor James Glass describes the atmosphere of Sheppard-Pratt Hospital while an SRA patient was being treated:"Suddenly books, police reports, compendia of newspaper articles on cults materialized; staff whispered in the hallways. . . . Many wondered if they should change their phone numbers or find dummy addresses or even take secret vacations from work, to throw off any would-be pursuers. People were careful whom they spoke with, and a few staff members refused to talk with me about anything to do with cults because they suspected that they and I were being 'watched.' " Finally even Glass succumbs: he starts to believe that his car is being followed, that the cult is breaking into his office, that a suspicious stranger at his undergraduate lecture is "a cult plant."[9] In Glass's view, it doesn't matter whether the terrors of SRA are real; but he overlooks his own evidence of the suggestibility of perfectly normal people to the paranoid hystories of satanic ritual abuse.

Benjamin, Bunny, and Scarlet: A Prototype

Who are the patients claiming satanic ritual abuse? In *Diagnosis for Disaster* (1995) Claudette Wassil-Grimm summarizes the prototype of an SRA patient. A woman goes to a therapist because of problems such as depression or bulimia. The therapist tells her she has symptoms that resemble those of childhood sexual abuse. She is "exhorted to read self-help books on incest, attend incest survivors' groups, and maybe attend an intensive weekend-long group therapy session." She begins to have vague memories of abuse. The memories grow. She sees many family neighbors involved—it must be satanic ritual abuse. "When she reports that she had a flashback of killing a baby and drinking the blood," the process of remembering is over. She can begin to recover, or "heal."[10] In a recent case that resembles the prototype, Connie Sievek started to see a psychotherapist for depression and remembered that she had seen her father and another man murder, disembowel, and bury a woman.[11] In another, "Tiffany Spencer" was branded, and her twin sister was sacrificed and dismembered.[12]

The third edition of *The Courage to Heal* (1994) adds a first-person narrative about MPD and ritual satanic abuse, which includes specifically Jewish imagery—significant, because many researchers have noted the link between SRA and the infamous "blood libel" of anti-Semitism, which goes back at least to the twelfth century.[13] It baffles researchers like Benjamin Beit-Hallahmi at the University of Haifa in Israel and Sherrill Mulhern in Paris that believers, many of whom are Jewish, ignore the connection between satanic narratives and traditional anti-Semitic lore. As Jeffrey S. Victor reminds us in *Satanic Panic: The Creation of a Contemporary Legend*, accusations of ritual child murder leveled at Jews reinforced beliefs "that Jews (like heretics) were in league with the Devil, that the Jews were agents of Satan on earth. . . . In the evolving Western demonology, the Devil was ultimately to blame for personal misfortune and social disaster. Therefore, the Jews, as the Devil's agents, could justly be punished for the pains of good and decent people."[14]

"S. R. Benjamin" is a Jewish biochemist in her forties with a Ph.D. from Yale. Her parents, she writes, belonged to a ring of child pornographers that also included a pediatrician, a psychologist, and an engineer. They used "pseudo-religious rituals with satanic overtones" to terrorize children, especially their own little daughter. Benjamin asserts she was auctioned into prostitution, witnessed the death of at least one child, and participated in the murder of a baby. She graphically describes being tortured with electricity and drugs, repeatedly raped by her father, and forced to sodomize her pet rabbit with a roofing nail. As a seventh grader, after her mother's death, she became pregnant and was compelled by her father and grandmother to undergo an abortion.

Benjamin was a prize-winning student who did not recall these horrifying experiences until 1986, when she was nearly through graduate school at Yale, married to a patient and supportive man, and having an extramarital affair. A veteran of many years of phobias and unsuccessful therapies, Benjamin attended a workshop for survivors of child abuse, and with dramatic suddenness the memories rose up. At Yale and then at Harvard, where she went for postdoctoral study, she remembered torture and began to present in therapy the three personalities she had developed to cope with it: "Benjamin—ageless, spiritual and protective; Bunny—little and worried; and Scarlet, the only female and the one who dealt with the sexual abuse." Benjamin's coworkers at Harvard were unsympathetic to her pain, tears, panics, and general dysfunction. She is still shocked by the "cruelty and scapegoating that most of the other postdoctoral fellows directed towards me," but she has forgiven them: they too may have been injured.

Despite her psychological difficulties, Benjamin finished her postdoctoral work and was hired as an assistant professor in a university research lab. There she began to recover memories of pornography and satanic rituals. She feels that she is finally coming to terms with her experience: "My history no longer defines me. It's something I've gone through, not who I am."

Like many of the names in *The Courage to Heal*, "S. R. Benjamin" is a pseudonym, but Bass and Davis tell us that her father, who belongs to the False Memory Syndrome Foundation, "vehemently denies that he ever abused his daughter in any way and has attributed his daughter's view of events to an irreversible psychosis."[15] Benjamin admits she is a phobic, self-mutilating, suicidal person who has panic attacks and carries around a lot of guilt. She relates this guilt to the possibility that she harmed other children through satanic rituals. She comforts herself with the thought that she was forced to commit these acts and that the crimes were possibly tricks, staged by the cult to keep her under control.

How has Benjamin managed to cope so well over the years? Can we believe that rape, abortion, child prostitution, even murder could have flourished undetected? Even Benjamin confesses to doubts about the truth of her account. But when a physical therapist explains away pains in her knees, she finds a more compliant physical therapist who validates her story. Benjamin says she reads about political torture, the Holocaust, Amnesty International, and satanic abuse. Watching an episode of *Star Trek* in which Commander Spock is tortured and broken yet retains his "competence and integrity" particularly inspires her.

Reading Benjamin's story as a hystory suggests that she is revealing her own sexual guilt and the puritanical values of her community, especially in relation to women. Nice Jewish girls are not supposed to be sexually titillated by the Holocaust or to betray decent husbands. Justifying such behavior to herself leads Benjamin to come up with a gigantic evil conspiracy. Having sexual feelings makes this otherwise docile intellectual feel so ashamed that she punishes herself—burns herself with cigarettes, feels suicidal. To exonerate and forgive herself, she imagines, imagines very vividly, that the sexuality comes from outside herself, from those stronger than she. Benjamin's family might have conveyed with unusual strength their disapproval of sexual behaviors. Could she have become pregnant in the seventh grade, when her mother died? Was there really an abortion, which left her feeling like a child murderer? Is this adolescent trauma the memory she cannot bear to face?

Jean La Fontaine has suggested that the common "motif of infant sacrifice in satanic rituals derives from anxiety and guilt about abortion."[16] But no warning bells go off for Bass and Davis. They consider satanic, or what they call sadistic, ritual abuse in the final section of *The Courage to Heal* and insist that the stories are not implausible. Readers who raise questions, they say, are in "collective denial." Implausibilities or inconsistencies in the narratives exist because the satanists deliberately confused things, "to lessen a survivor's credibility should she or he seek help." Bass and Davis invoke the Talmud in asking people to confront these horrors.[17] English therapist Valerie Sinason also compares SRA denial with Holocaust denial.[18]

SRA and Gender

It should come as no surprise that most adults recovering memories of SRA are women. Leslie Bennetts writes that psychiatrists explain that "traumatized women tend to turn up in the mental-health system while men with similar histories act out, often in violent ways, and end up in jail."[19]

Women also dominate the SRA subculture—that is, the people who have been most upset by allegations of satanic ritual abuse. Journalist Debbie Nathan and lawyer Michael Snedeker, who co-authored *Satan's Silence: Ritual Abuse and the Making of a Modern American Witch Hunt* (1995), suggest that "being a ritual-abuse victim's parent is a feminine role. 'Believing the children,' in other words, is women's work." They add that "mothers become far more involved in the cases, doing everything from shuttling their children to therapy, to attending support groups, to trekking day after day to court." Nathan and Snedeker hypothesize that outrage about alleged SRA allows women a sanctioned outlet for frustrations and angers otherwise ignored. More mothers of children in SRA cases sought counseling than fathers did, and these women used the therapy "to consider matters that had troubled them for years, but which they were only able to deal with now because they linked them to their children's victimization." They often complained about indifferent or demanding husbands; some said they withdrew sexually from their husbands after the children's alleged abuse. Many couples separated or divorced. "Ritual abuse," Nathan and Snedeker conclude, "thus helped women disengage from unsatisfactory marriages without feeling guilty about being bad wives or mothers. After all, the reason they weren't getting along with their husbands was because they cared so much about their children."[20]

SRA and Feminism

Feminist therapists, activists, and academics have been entangled in the SRA dispute, as they have in other areas of the recovered memory movement—especially in England, where they have played a leading role as theorists. According to Nathan and Snedeker, "Feminists were particularly susceptible to sex-abuse conspiracy theories."[21] In the feminist journal *SIGNS* in 1993, Linda Alcoff and Laura Gray, two Syracuse University professors, compare the testimony of ritual abuse with testimony of rape victims who may not be believed: "Survivors of especially heinous ritualized sexual abuse are not believed. The pattern that emerges from these disparate responses is that if survivor speech is not silenced before it is uttered, it is categorized within the mad, the untrue, or the incredible."[22]

Ironically, the SRA panic derives in large part from religious fundamentalists and political conservatives who are antagonistic to feminist goals. By the late 1980s, Nathan and Snedeker declare, "opponents of state involvement in family life were using ritual-abuse accusations as a warning about the dangers of child protection and therapy, and issuing across-the-board condemnations of feminism and feminists as predatory wreckers of happy homes. Ritual-abuse proponents responded by dismissing every criticism as antifeminist and antichild backlash, all the while ignoring their own complicity in discrediting child protection and the women's movement."[23]

Nathan and Snedeker deplore the alliance between such feminists as Gloria Steinem and "a moral crusade engaged in dangerous flirtation with antiabortionists, homophobes, racists, and proponents of the principle that a woman's place is in the home. . . . Indeed, during the past decade, belief in ritual abuse has become so ensconced in this wing of feminism that the arrest, trial by ordeal, and lifelong incarceration of accused women have occasioned hardly a blink from its proponents. They have remained silent as convicted mothers and teachers are sent to prison."[24]

Telling Satanic Stories

Why do so many intelligent, educated, concerned people believe these bizarre stories? The term *satanic ritual abuse* is a large and messy one that can be stretched to cover several phenomena; its vagueness and inclusiveness make it seem plausible to many reasonable people who recall having read or heard something that may relate to it. Although advocates frequently compare SRA with the Manson murders or the Jim Jones mass suicides in Guyana, followers of Manson or Jones were not masked as ordinary upstanding citizens. Child molesters, pornographers, and child sex rings exemplify real abuse that has no documented connection to satanism. Marginalized teenagers playing heavy metal music and tattooing themselves with skulls may alarm adults, but they are not the transgenerational secret satanists of rumor.

Language plays a role as well. Therapists speak of "satanic ritual abuse" rather than "alleged satanic ritual abuse which has never been proven or corroborated." "The result," writes Sherrill Mulhern, "is that by the magic of language, ritual abuse suddenly appears. We are talking about it as if it had some objective meaning outside of the subjective meanings that each individual . . . attributes to the terms. This confers an aura of reality on phenomena which may or may not have ever occurred."[25]

Finally, SRA is a way of dealing with horrifying human pathologies. Jean La Fontaine writes that "a belief in evil cults is convincing because it draws on powerful cultural axioms. People are reluctant to accept that parents, even those classed as social failures, will harm their own children, and even invite others to do so, but involvement with the devil explains it. The notion that unknown, powerful leaders control the cult revives an old myth of dangerous strangers. Demonising the marginal poor and linking them to unknown satanists turns intractable cases of abuse into manifestations of evil."

Hystories of SRA are flexible and creative. When basic practical questions are asked, details of the satanic narrative shift. If a patient claims to have seen babies murdered and buried but the police can find no bodies, the therapist explains that the patient had been hypnotically programmed to conceal the site, or that she was afraid to expose the real perpetrators, or that the cult had duped her into believing a crime had been committed so that she would not be believed in the future.[26] If bodies cannot be found, patients sometimes allege that the satanists ate or burned them. If police explain that ordinary fire is not hot enough to totally destroy a body, patients tell stories of special industrial furnaces.

SRA advocates defend the consistency of the narratives but seem not to understand the power of literary conventions, the morphology of folk tales, the repetition of rumors, and above all the way that suggestion works to produce confabulation. At conferences and seminars therapists are exhorted to believe. They hear emotional testimony from "survivors," followed by standing ovations. All the sensational theater that worked so well at the Salpêtrière is put to use on the SRA conference circuit. Patients learn to tell their stories too. Sherrill Mulhern, who has looked at transcripts, says that "initially, patients were not saying the same things but came to say similar things over time." Memories of satanic rituals develop slowly after a patient has spent a lot of time in therapy: "They begin as isolated images and/or affects—distributed over a number of different personalities—which must be gradually identified and pieced together." The "satanism" of the satanic ritual abuse narratives, Mulhern concludes, is "essentially a rehashing of the satanic confabulations of a variety of individuals, which have been homogenized into a single Satanism through hours of networking between therapists, Satan investigators, and survivors."[27] Therapists elicit memories by asking patients questions about a long list of items, by focusing on vague feelings, by giving shape and meaning to fragments.

Even when they describe the cultural source of satanic images, however, many therapists seem not to recognize its influence. They quote Tolkein, or describe a movie called *The Witches* (1966), in which Joan Fontaine plays a school teacher who stumbles upon a secret coven, or draw attention to the popularity of movies about devils, witchcraft, and possession. Others quote medieval studies of witchcraft as if they were finding historical evidence rather than plot motifs in folk lore and popular religion. Yet, says George Greaves, "no single book or movie contains the material of even a single patient."[28]

Ira Levin's best-selling novel *Rosemary's Baby* (1967), made into a hit film starring Mia Farrow in 1968, remains a significant source for the details and decor of much SRA narrative. The movie had unusual cultural power because the wife of director Roman Polanski was herself murdered by the Charles Manson cult—an event that drew worldwide publicity. The diabolist of the novel, also named Roman, leads a satanic cult that makes a deal with Guy, a struggling young actor; he will find success and fame if he helps them trick his wife, Rosemary, into bearing Satan's child. Rosemary begins to have suspicions of her neighbors and does research on witchcraft: "They use *blood* in their rituals, because blood has *power*, and the blood that has the *most* power is a *baby's* blood, a baby that hasn't been baptized, and they use *more* than the blood, they use the *flesh* too!" Despite her struggles, Rosemary has the baby, which she beholds in a black bassinet, wrapped in a black blanket, surrounded by black candles and black-wrapped presents. She decides to cooperate with the cult, and to raise her child.

Rosemary's Doctors

Novels and movies create popular imagery, but satanic ritual abuse stories can't flourish unless therapists are willing to stake their reputations on the cases. In the United States, distinguished therapists who have taken SRA seriously respond to the call for clear-headed investigation of the evidence with passionate claims that they are healers, not law enforcement officers. "I'm a psychology person," Dan Sexton of the National Child Abuse Hot Line said in 1989, "so I don't need the evidence."[29]

SRA therapists have themselves been at the center of lawsuits and exposés. Judith Peterson, a therapist at Spring Shadows Glen in Houston, has been sued by seven patients. Another controversial therapist, Bennett Braun, hospitalized Mary Shanley, a thirty-nine-year-old primary school teacher. Although she disliked Braun, Shanley was impressed by his colleague Roberta Sachs. Medicated with Inderal, Xanax, Prozac, Klonopin, and Halcion, among other tranquilizers, SSRIs, beta blockers, and sedatives, Shanley believed she had been trained by her mother to be the high priestess of a satanic cult: "I remembered going to rituals and witnessing sacrifices. I had a baby at age 13, supposedly, and that child was sacrificed." After a workshop with Cory Hammond, Shanley and her husband were persuaded that her nine-year-old son should also be treated or the cult would kill him. Shanley was sent to Spring Shadows Glen under the care of Judith Peterson.[30]

In a "Frontline" TV documentary called "The Search for Satan," produced by Ofra Bike and Rachel Dretzin, Shanley, called "Mary S.," told her story. The program suggested a financial motive behind the cases: MPD and SRA patients are often covered by "very rich benefit plans." Mary S.'s insurance company paid more than $2.5 million for her treatment, and a nurse testified that the unit at Spring Shadows Glen Hospital was "very profitable."[31] Peterson, now in private practice, has hired lawyers to defend her against patients' allegations and file counter-suits. She sees herself, Mark Pendergrast reports, as "an altruistic, idealistic person trying to help the world. She started her career working with migrant workers and Head Start children and parents." In Peterson's view, *she* is the victim of her patients: "The shame and guilt were then transferred to me, the therapist. Kill the messenger. Lie. This client relieved the trauma by victimizing me. Suddenly, the therapist is the victim."[32]

Professor Cory Hammond of the University of Utah Medical School has long maintained that satanic cults are part of a Nazi conspiracy led by a renegade Jew. Hammond, a psychologist and specialist in hypnosis, has been teaching and lecturing about satanic abuse for many years, despite his stated fears that the cults will assassinate him for betraying their secrets. At a meeting of the Fourth Annual Regional Conference on Abuse and Multiple Personality Disorder in 1992, he declared that satanic cults in the United States are masterminded by a Jewish doctor named Green, originally Greenbaum. As a teenager in Germany, Green collaborated with satanic Nazi scientists, helped by his knowledge of the Kabala. Once in the United States, he joined forces with the CIA to work on brainwashing and mind control. Hammond believes that Green's satanic cults intend to create "tens of thousands of mental robots who will do pornography, prostitution, smuggle drugs, and engage in international arms smuggling. Eventually, those at the top of the satanic cult want to create a satanic order that will rule the world."[33]

Hammond describes how the programming of children begins when they are two or three. They are strapped down, hooked up to an intravenous supply of Demoral, and connected to electrodes; the programmers use electric shocks to reinforce their message. Hammond's description of alter personalities sounds like Huxley's *Brave New World*:

> Alpha represents general programming. Beta appears to be sexual programs, such as how to perform oral sex in a certain way or how to produce and direct child pornography films or run child prostitution rings. Delta are killers. Delta-alters are trained

to kill in ceremonies and also do some self-harm stuff. Theta are psychic killers. This comes from their belief in psychic abilities including their belief that they can make someone develop a brain tumor and die. Omega are self-destruct programs which can make the patient self-mutilate or kill themselves. Gamma systems are protection and deception programs which provide misinformation to try and misdirect you. There are also other Greek letter programs. Zeta has to do with the production of snuff films. Omicron has to do with their association with the Mafia, big business, and government leaders.[34]

In Hammond's view, cult members control these robots with laptop computers and activate them with hand signals. He believes that the program can also be activated by reciting an erasure code to the patient. "When you give the code and ask what the patient is experiencing, they will describe computers whirring, things erasing and things exploding and vaporizing." In his communication with patients under hypnosis, Hammond uses finger signals to elicit agreement. Patients have virtually no verbal input; all is appropriated and incorporated into Hammond's hystory—a singularly detailed, anti-Semitic, and scary one. When asked about the absence of evidence, Hammond responds, "The things that therapists hear all over this country are that morticians are involved in many cases, physicians who can sign phony death certificates."[35]

England too has therapist-advocates who believe in horrific conspiracies, such as Joan Coleman, associate specialist in Psychiatry at Healthlands Mental Health Services in Surrey. In 1989 Dr. Coleman, an "expert" on the structure of satanic cults, organized RAINS, the Ritual Abuse Information Network and Support. Coleman's first SRA patient described witnessing the ritual abuse and murder of three Vietnamese children in 1967. In her story, the ritual involved classic paraphernalia of the witches sabbath—candles, inverted crosses, robes, and masks. Satanists drank blood from a chalice and practiced cannibalism: "Much of the children's flesh was eaten prior to the remains being burnt." Coleman expresses her horror at the story, but apparently didn't ask her patient how these children, described as "among the first contingent of 'boat people' brought to Southampton from the USA," could have traveled such an odd and circuitous route to England and then disappeared without any publicity. Coleman's second SRA patient recounted stories of feral, retarded, or traumatized children hanging in cages in the basement of a house, "brought out only for abuse or experimental operations performed by the cult leader, who, she thought, was a doctor."[36] Coleman offers no evidence of the truth of this appalling story.

Coleman calls SRA "a way of life," with children indoctrinated at home by their mothers. She provides an elaborate outline of the hierarchical structure of cults, which include prominent and distinguished members of the community—doctors, lawyers, politicians, clergy, and ambassadors, as well as members of the upper class. The basic unit is the thirteen-person Coven, which gathers into larger groups of circles or lodges headed by high priests or priestesses. In their religious rituals, the Covens worship Satan through weekly or holiday festivals, using clothing and ceremonies that parody Christian ritual, and practice human sacrifice. Children in the cults must submit to intense brainwashing and mind control. They are given talismanic objects or poppets; some also remember operations in which a surveillance device was implanted, to punish them if they betrayed the cult. (Among Valerie Sinason's patients, Jane had to kill and eat her pet budgie; Rita found her slaughtered dog in her bed; Malcolm had to lie on a female corpse.)[37] Children are regularly sexually abused by parents and priests or priestesses. Some of the abuse involves electric shocks, and Christian symbols are often part of the ritual.

Coleman mentions "poppets" as if she never heard of *The Crucible*, in which the poppet planted in the home of one of the accused is such an important plot device. The range, detail, and credulity of Coleman's list—all of it without the least scrap of evidence—is shocking. Like other therapists, she has worked out an elaborate system to explain the absence of substantiating evidence. The big stuff, like altars, is concealed in members' garages. Ritual objects, like the goats' heads and daggers, are kept in "shops selling military memorabilia or antiques." The evil books are locked up in safes. Tarpaulins cover traces of blood. Corpses are buried, sunk in rivers, burned in furnaces or crematoria, dissolved in acid baths, minced in machines, fed to dogs and pigs, or eaten by the coven. Victims come from anonymous populations: runaways from deprived families who have not reported them missing, aborted fetuses, children of cult members, vagrants, and renegades.

Cult members apparently have to keep up with their busy public careers as well as running around to coven meetings, doing their share of molesting, and getting rid of bodies through time-consuming and elaborate methods. Why do they put up with such a life? Coleman responds that those at the top of the heap make vast sums from extortion and child pornography and prostitution rings, maybe even a little arms dealing. Those on the bottom are bribed with money to pay off their mortgages, take holidays, or buy new cars and "string-pulling to further their careers, sometimes with the aid of Masonic connections."[38]

Joan Coleman was predictably unhappy with the La Fontaine report. In a letter to the *London Review of Books*, she pointed to the internal consistency in stories from unrelated sources and to the inexplicable weirdness of male professional behavior: "Personally, I, too, have difficulty with the concept of satanic worship and I am no nearer to believing in black or any other sort of magic than I ever was, but it's almost equally hard to understand how grown men, mostly from the professional classes, can go along with the extraordinary initiation rites involved in Freemasonry."[39]

The most distinguished advocate of SRA in England is Valerie Sinason, consultant child psychotherapist at the Tavistock Clinic, who has edited an influential book called *Treating Survivors of Satanist Sexual Abuse*. Many of my friends in the London psychiatric community urged me to meet Sinason (I did not) and assured me that I would like and respect her. Her peers regard her as a skilled clinician who has done exemplary work with mentally handicapped patients, including adults who have a mental age of less than eight (and therefore have no legal rights to testify in English courts). Sinason regards herself as the advocate of severely handicapped patients—patients few therapists are willing to treat. Like the clinicians who developed automatic writing with Ouija boards for autistic patients but did not consciously know that they themselves were transmitting messages, guiding the planquettes, Sinason denies projecting abuse and satanism onto her patients. Leslie Wilson, who interviewed Sinason for the *London Review of Books*, says that she "has the intensity of the embattled campaigner rather than the obsessional quality of a zealot."

Sinason has staked her professional reputation on belief in satanic ritual abuse. It would be more than awkward for her to back down. When the English government's report found no evidence to support claims of devil worship in eighty-four cases, Sinason stuck to her guns, telling the press that although some people might have satanist fantasies, abuse really existed.[40] "If you see people you care about not getting justice," she told Leslie Wilson, "it is your duty to bring that to the attention of the proper structure."[41]

Sinason's introduction to the English edition of Lawrence Wright's *Remembering Satan* is a vivid instance of her skill in negotiating the borders between scientific objectivity and her own convictions about SRA. Wright is a journalist whose investigation of the Ingram family case in Olympia, Washington, had a huge impact in 1993 when it appeared in the *New Yorker*. In 1988 Paul Ingram's two teenage daughters accused him of abuse and implicated the whole family of conservative fundamentalists, as well as many other people, in satanic ritualism. Ingram, a devout churchman, went along with the accusations. He recanted too late and was sentenced to twenty years in prison. Lawrence Wright's thoughtful, thorough, and compassionate study of the case alerted Americans to the dangers of recovered memory and religious fundamentalism. Persuading Wright to accept an introduction written by Valerie Sinason and persuading Sinason to write a respectful introduction to a book that, if taken seriously, discredits everything she has been doing was no mean task for the editors at Serpent's Tail, a small radical press based in London.

But the introduction is a small masterpiece of evasion. Sinason appears at first to acknowledge the justice of Wright's argument, calling *Remembering Satan* a "highly significant, intelligent book which raises serious concerns."[42] But this superficial flexibility soon disappears in a thicket of conditional "if" clauses and passive impersonal constructions. On the rhetorical level, Sinason tries to eat her cake and have it too—"if" Wright is correct, *then* a "serious injustice has been unwittingly perpetrated on one family." The identity of the perpetrators? Unnamed. Did they have any control over their acts? No, they behaved "unwittingly." The phrase "one family" is important too. Sinason concedes, perhaps, a single mistake but insists that cases of mistaken accusations are rare and unimportant compared to the enormity of abuse. There are more "real incidents" than complaints of false accusation. She cites a colleague's "cautious estimate" that 15 to 30 percent of all sixteen-year-old girls have suffered some kind of sexual abuse, much of it incestuous.

In defending her position, Sinason tries to present the issue as one of different opinions or different perspectives or different interests or different interpretations or different conclusions. She pleads for tolerance of others' opinions, for "different ways of seeing," and asserts that the absence of hard evidence matters less than the concern expressed by clinicians who have heard the stories of abuse. These trained clinicians, Sinason writes, "were far more likely to accurately perceive behaviour linked to abuse," but she offers no real evidence of this assumption, nor a definition of what "accurate" means.

Out of Darkness: The Dangers of SRA

Is satanic ritual abuse a fad diagnosis or a sign of social danger? Mulhern calls the satanism scare "a rumor in search of an inquisition."[43] Newspaper accounts see the rumor as a clear sequence of events and epidemic contagion. Like stories of the genesis of AIDS, the narratives often point to a single source or mediating figure, a Satanist Patient X. Journalists also seek to pin blame for the epidemic on an external source. The London *Times*, for example, blames Americans: "Influence by American Christian fundamentalists led to allegations of satanic abuse surfacing in Britain in the late 1980s. The term originated in America after the publication in 1980 of *Michelle Remembers* by Lawrence Pazder, a psychiatrist, which told the story of a girl being ritually abused by satanists, one of whom was her mother." According to the newspaper, the term "caught on in Britain when Pamela Klein, who worked at a rape crisis center at Southern Illinois University, moved here in 1985." Mrs. Klein "organized a conference on child abuse at Reading University in 1989, and theories of satanic abuse spread among social workers."[44] Under the headline "Beast that runs wild in US imagination," another *Times* journalist wrote, "The mythical beast known as satanic sex abuse was born in America, where it has all the hallmarks of a panic craze fed by films, television and books, nurtured by fantasy, maintained by a plethora of accusations and bolstered by the credulity of psychotherapists and the public."[45] English journalists have denounced satanic ritual abuse as a kind of "American social disease."

But the reality is more complicated. Michelle was actually Canadian, and English satanist theories come from several independent sources. Indeed, as Bryan Appleyard recognized in a 1994 essay, "Who the Devil Shall We Blame?" in *The Independent*, "Satan was always a metaphor for what is inside, not what is outside." Despite the human tendency to locate evil fantasies outside the self, they reflect impulses within all individuals and cultures. English or American, until we can accept that truth, we have not outlived Satan's dark legacy.

In the courts, satanic abuse accusations are now facing more skeptical juries. In December 1995, Robert and Constance Roberson, a lay pastor and his wife from Wenatchee, Washington, were acquitted of

charges that they led a sex ring in which children were raped and ritually abused. "There was nothing to this case," a juror told the *New York
Times*. "Why did they bring this to trial? Here were all these people
who had attended every church service for the past three or four years,
who had never seen anything like what the prosecution was describing, and their prosecutors had never even talked to them."[46] More than
a dozen verdicts have been overturned since 1990, and Linda Fairstein,
chief of the Manhattan District Attorney's sex crimes unit, calls mass-
molestation cases "the most flawed class of prosecutions ever."[47]

Yet many others who have been accused remain imprisoned.
Rather than accept the lack of evidence for their claims, many patients, therapists, and believers have expanded their definitions of
abuse, as Debbie Nathan and Michael Snedeker observe, "replacing the
term *satanic* with *sadistic* and lengthening the list of possible conspira-
tors to include more traditional social devils such as the KKK, the neo-
Nazis, the survivalists, marginal religious cults, and the brainwashing
enthusiasts of the CIA."[48] Their fascination with conspiracy bodes ill for
the prospect that we will soon emerge from this darkness. Kenneth
Lanning cautions "overzealous intervenors" that relentless publicity
can exacerbate the problem: "Are we encouraging needy or traumatized individuals to tell more and more outrageous tales of their victimization? Are we now making up for centuries of denial by blindly
accepting any allegation of child abuse no matter how absurd or
unlikely?"[49] The answers to these questions over the next few years
will determine whether SRA rumors become hysterical inquisition or
just historical curiosities.

16. Albert D. Vandam, "The Trail of 'Trilby,'" *The Forum* 20 (September 1895–February 1896): 434–35.

17. See Ulrich Baer, "Photography and Hysteria: Towards a Poetics of the Flash," *Yale Journal of Criticism*, 7 (1994): 66ff.

18. Goldstein, *Console and Classify*, 330.

19. Ellenberger, "Charcot and the Salpêtrière School," 150.

20. Evans, *Fits and Starts*, 41.

21. Mark S. Micale, "On the 'Disappearance' of Hysteria: A Study in the Clinical Deconstruction of a Diagnosis," *Isis*, 84 (1993): 525.

22. Paul Dubois, *The Psychic Treatment of Nervous Disorders*, Eng. trans., 6th ed. (New York, 1909), 15–16, quoted in Shorter, *From Paralysis to Fatigue*, 185.

23. Micale, "On the 'Disappearance' of Hysteria," 89.

24. A. Steyerthal, *Was ist Hysterie?*, quoted in Webster, *Why Freud Was Wrong* (New York: Basic Books, 1995), 138.

25. Micale, "On the 'Disappearance' of Hysteria," 500.

26. Ibid., 501.

27. Webster, *Why Freud Was Wrong*, 9.

28. John Forrester and Lisa Appignanesi, *Freud's Women* (New York: Basic Books, 1993), 71.

29. For a provocative discussion of the importance of this case, see Dianne Hunter, "Hysteria, Psychoanalysis, and Feminism: The Case of Anna O.," *Feminist Studies*, 9 (Fall 1983): 465–88.

30. Sigmund Freud, *An Autobiographical Study* [1925] (New York: Norton, 1952), 33.

31. *The Complete Letters of Sigmund Freud to Wilhelm Fliess*, ed. Jeffrey Moussaief Masson (Cambridge: Harvard University Press, 1985), 212.

32. Jeffrey Moussaief Masson, *The Assault on Truth: Freud's Suppression of the Seduction Theory* (New York: Farrar Straus Giroux, 1984), xv–xxiii.

33. Judith Lewis Herman, *Father-Daughter Incest* (Cambridge: Harvard University Press, 1981), 10.

34. Masson, *The Assault on Truth*, 144.

35. See Richard Webster, "The Seduction Theory," in *Why Freud Was Wrong*, 195–213.

36. Frederick Crews, *The Memory Wars: Freud's Legacy in Dispute* (New York: New York Review Books, 1995), 59.

37. Webster, *Why Freud Was Wrong*, 213.

38. Sigmund Freud, *Dora: An Analysis of a Case of Hysteria* (New York: Collins, 1964), 20. See also Charles Bernheimer and Claire Kahane, eds., *In Dora's Case: Freud-Hysteria-Feminism* (New York: Columbia University Press, 1985).

39. Jeffrey M. Masson, *Against Therapy* (London: Fontana, 1990), 101.

40. Kurt Eissler, "The Effect of the Structure of the Ego in Psychoanalytic Technique," *Journal of the American Psychoanalytic Association*, 1 (1953): 114.

41. Juliet Mitchell, "The Question of Femininity and the Theory of Psychoanalysis," in *The British School of Psychoanalysis*, ed. Gregorio Kohon (London: Free Association Books, 1986), 386.

42. Evans, *Fits and Starts*, 2.

43. Frederick Crews, "The Unknown Freud," *New York Review of Books*, November 18, 1993, 55.

44. Frederick Crews, letter to the editor, *New York Times*, December 13, 1995, A22.

45. Sebastian Faulks, "Freudian Snips," *The Guardian*, October 31, 1995, 6.

46. Sherry Turkle, *Psychoanalytic Politics: Jacques Lacan and Freud's French Revolution* (New York: Basic Books, 1978; London: Burnett Books, 1979), 14.

47. Elisabeth Roudinesco, *Jacques Lacan & Co.*, trans. Jeffrey Mehlman (Chicago: University of Chicago Press, 1990), 420.

48. Evans, *Fits and Starts*, 174.

49. André Breton and Louis Aragon, "Le cinquantenaire de l'hystérie, 1878–1928," in Breton, *Oeuvres complètes* (Paris: Gallimard, 1988), 1:948–50.

50. Catherine Clément, *The Lives and Legends of Jacques Lacan* (New York: Columbia University Press, 1983), 12, 55.

51. Mark S. Micale and Roy Porter, eds. *Discovering the History of Psychiatry* (New York/Oxford: Oxford University Press, 1994), 13.

52. See Stuart A. Kirk and Herb Kutchins, *The Selling of DSM: The Rhetoric of Science in Psychiatry* (New York: Aldine de Gruyter, 1992), 8.

4. Politics, Patients, and Feminism

1. Judith Lewis Herman, *Trauma and Recovery* (New York: Basic Books, 1992), 32.

2. William Barry, "The Strike of a Sex," *Quarterly Review*, 179 (1894): 312.

3. Lisa Tickner, *The Spectacle of Women* (Chicago: University of Chicago Press, 1988), 315n188.

4. Fritz Wittels, *Die Fackel*, May 1907, quoted in Hannah S. Decker, *Freud, Dora, and Vienna 1900* (New York, The Free Press, 1991), 201.

5. S. Weir Mitchell, *Doctor and Patient* (Philadelphia: Lippincott, 1888), 48.

6. John Forrester and Lisa Appignanesi, *Freud's Women* (New York: Basic Books, 1993), 68.

7. See Elizabeth Lunbeck, *The Psychiatric Persuasion* (Princeton: Princeton University Press, 1994), 209–28.

8. "Sof'ia Niron" (pseud.), in *Russkie vedemosti* 1 (November 1888), rpt S. V. Kovalevskaia, *Vospominaniia Povesti* (Moscow: Izdatel'stvo Nauka, 1974), 275–81. Thanks to Prof. Debora Silverman, History Department, UCLA, for this reference.

9. Georgette Déga, *Essai sur la cure préventive de l'hystérie féminine par l'éducation* (Paris: Alcan, 1898), 24, 26.

10. Martha Noel Evans, *Fits and Starts: A Genealogy of Hysteria in Modern France* (Ithaca: Cornell University Press, 1991), 73.

11. Nancy Chodorow, *Feminism and Psychoanalytic Theory* (New Haven: Yale University Press, 1989), 199–218.

12. Chodorow, *Feminism and Psychoanalytic Theory*, 208–10.

13. Forrester and Appignanesi, *Freud's Women*, 319.

14. Chodorow, *Feminism and Psychoanalytic Theory*, 213, 217.

15. Carroll Smith-Rosenberg, "The Hysterical Woman: Sex Roles and Role Conflict in Nineteenth-Century America," *Social Research*, 39 (1972): 652–78. Reprinted in Smith-Rosenberg, *Disorderly Conduct: Visions of Gender in Victorian America* (New York: Knopf, 1985), 197–216.

16. Mark Pendergrast, *Victims of Memory: Incest Accusations and Shattered Lives* (Hinesburg, Vt.: Upper Access, 1995), 429.

17. Nancy Tomes, "Feminist History of Psychiatry," in Mark S. Micale and Roy Porter, eds., *Discovering the History of Psychiatry* (New York/Oxford: Oxford University Press, 1994), 358.

18. Evans, *Fits and Starts*, 205

19. Ibid., 203–4.

20. Ibid., 215.

21. Hélène Cixous, "Sorties," in *The Newly Born Woman*, trans. Betsy Wing (Minneapolis: University of Minnesota Press, 1975), 99.

22. Evans, *Fits and Starts*, 210.

23. Claire Kahane, "Introduction: Part Two," *In Dora's Case: Freud-Hysteria-Feminism*, Charles Bernheimer and Claire Kahane, eds. (New York: Columbia University Press, 1985), 27.

24. Mandy Merck, "The Critical Cult of *Dora*," in Merck, *Perversions* (London: Virago, 1993), 33–44.

25. Mark S. Micale, *Approaching Hysteria* (Princeton: Princeton University Press, 1994), 84.

26. Janet Malcolm, "Reflections: J'appelle un chat un chat," *In Dora's Case*, 2d ed., 305.

27. Dianne Hunter, "Hysteria, Psychoanalysis, and Feminism: The Case of Anna O.," *Feminist Studies*, 9 (Fall 1983): 484.

28. Diane Price Herndl, "The Writing Cure," *NWSA Journal*, 1 (1988): 53.

29. See Ilene J. Philipson, *On the Shoulders of Women: The Feminization of Psychotherapy* (New York/London: Guilford Press, 1993), 54–55.

30. Ibid., 114, 116, 148.

31. Ellen Bass and Laura Davis, *The Courage to Heal*, 3d ed. (New York: Harper Perennial, 1994), 482.

32. Ian Hacking, *Rewriting the Soul: Multiple Personality and the Sciences of Memory* (Princeton: Princeton University Press, 1995), 62.

33. Judith Lewis Herman, *Father-Daughter Incest* (Cambridge: Harvard University Press, 1981), 29.

34. Laura S. Brown, "Not Outside the Range: One Feminist Perspective on Psychic Trauma," in *Trauma: Explorations in Memory*, ed. Cathy Carruth (Baltimore: Johns Hopkins University Press, 1995), 102–3.

35. Maria P. Root, "Reconstructing the Impact of Trauma on Personality," in *Personality and Psychopathology: Feminist Reappraisals*, ed. L. S. Brown and M. Baillou (New York: Guilford, 1992).

36. Carol Tavris, *The Mismeasure of Woman* (New York: Simon and Schuster, 1992), 321.

5. Hysterical Men

1. S. Weir Mitchell, "A Case of Uncomplicated Hysteria in the Male," unpublished manuscript in Philadelphia College of Medicine, 1904.

2. Mark S. Micale, "Hysteria Male/Hysteria Female," in *Science and Sensibility*, ed. Marina Benjamin (London: Basil Blackwell, 1991), 3.

3. Pierre Marie, "Eloge de J.-M. Charcot," *Bulletin de l'Académie de Médicine*, 93 (1925): 576–93, quoted in Georges Guillain, *J.-M. Charcot, 1825–1893: His Life*, trans. Pearce Bailey (London: Pitman Medical, 1959), 146.

4. See J.-M. Charcot, *Clinical Lectures on Diseases of the Nervous System*, Ruth Harris, ed. (New York/London: Tavistock, 1991). Charcot's major lectures on male hysteria were originally published in *Oeuvres completes de J-M Charcot*, 9 vols. (Paris: Bureau de Progrès Medical, Delahaye et Lecosnier, 1886–1893).

5. Robert Brudenell Carter, *On the Pathology and Treatment of Hysteria* (London: Churchill, 1853), 34.

6. Thomas Laycock, *A Treatise on the Nervous Diseases of Women* (1840), quoted by Janet Oppenheim, *Shattered Nerves: Doctors, Patients, and Depression in Victorian England* (New York: Oxford University Press, 1991), 143.

7. Ernst von Feuchtersleben, *The Principles of Medical Psychology* (1847), quoted in Ilza Veith, *Hysteria: The History of a Disease* (Chicago: University of Chicago Press, 1965), 169.

8. "Un mécanicien de locomotive hystérique! Un homme fort, solide, habitué aux intempéries des saisons, est-ce raisonnable? On peut s'imaginer une femmelette parfumée et pommadée souffrant de ce mal bizarre; mais qu'un ouvrier robuste ait ses nerfs et des vapeurs comme une dame de grand monde, c'est trop!" Emile Batault, *Contribution à l'étude de l'hystérie chez l'homme* (Paris, 1885), 48.

9. Jean-Martin Charcot, quoted in Jan Goldstein, *Console and Classify: The French Psychiatric Profession in the Nineteenth Century* (New York: Cambridge University Press, 1987), 336.

10. Brian Donkin, quoted in Oppenheim, *Shattered Nerves*, 144, 115.

11. F. S. Gosling, *Before Freud: Neurasthenia and the American Medical Community* (Urbana: Illinois University Press, 1987), 47.

12. Archibald Church, quoted in Gosling, *Before Freud*, 115, and Oppenheim, *Shattered Nerves*, 144.

13. See "The Railway God," in George Frederick Drinka, *The Birth of Neurosis: Myth, Malady, and the Victorians* (New York: Simon & Schuster, 1983), 108–22.

14. Jean-Martin Charcot, quoted in Mark S. Micale, "J.-M. Charcot and the Idea of Hysteria in the Male," *Medical History*, 34 (October 1990), 25.

15. Paul Fabre, "De l'hystérie chez l'homme," *Gazette médicale Paris*, 3 (December 3, 1881): 867.

16. Charcot, "Six Cases of Hysteria in the Male," in *Clinical Lectures on*

Diseases of the Nervous System, ed. Ruth Harris (London: Routledge, 1991), 236–42.

17. Charcot, "Des propensités hystéro-traumatiques chez l'homme," *Semaine médicale*, 7 (1887): 491.

18. Charcot, *Leçons du mardi*, 2:50

19. Jules Déjerine, quoted in Micale, "Charcot and the Idea of Hysteria in the Male," 36.

20. Charcot, "Six Cases," 236–42.

21. Ruth Harris, "Introduction," *Clinical Lectures*, xxxiii.

22. Charcot, "Six Cases," 236–42.

23. Emile Batault, *Contribution à l'étude de l'hystérie chez l'homme*, 110.

24. Charcot, "Six Cases," 239.

25. J.-M. Charcot, "Hystérie et dégénérescence chez l'homme," in' Etienne Trillat, ed., *L'hystérie* (Toulouse: Edouard Privat, 1971), 143–53 (my translation).

26. On the astonishing iconography of tattoos among *28 million* male prisoners and Soviet labor camps in the Soviet republics, see Arkady G. Bonnikov, "Body Language," *New York Times*, November 6, 1993, 23.

27. Michèle Ouerd, "Introduction," Charcot, *Leçons sur l'hystérie virile* (Paris: Le Sycamore, 1984), 27.

28. Goldstein, *Console and Classify*, 154.

29. Cyril Burt, *The Subnormal Mind* (Oxford: Oxford University Press, 1977), 5.

30. Philip Gibbs, in Eric Leed, *No Man's Land: Combat and Identity in World War I* (Cambridge: Cambridge University Press, 1979), 187.

31. Ibid., 185.

32. See Oswald Bumke and Hans Burger-Prinz, *Ein Psychiater berichter* (Hamburg: Hoffman und Campe, 1971), 102, trans. Edward Shorter in *From Paralysis to Fatigue* (New York: The Free Press, 1992), 271.

33. P. LeFebvre and S. Barbass, "L'hystérie de guerre: Etude comparative de ses manifestations au cours des derniers conflits mondiaux," *Annales médico-psychologiques*, 142 (1984): 262–66, quoted in Shorter, *Paralysis and Fatigue*, 265.

34. Martin Blumenson, *Patton: The Man Behind the Legend* (New York: Morrow, 1985), 210–11.

35. See Nathan G. Hale, Jr., *The Rise and Crisis of Psychoanalysis in the United States* (New York: Oxford University Press, 1995), 276–81.

36. Zahava Solomon, *Combat Stress Reaction: The Enduring Toll of War* (New York: Plenum Press, 1993), vii, 163.

37. See Richard A. Kuhl et al., *Trauma and the Vietnam War Generation* (New York: Brunner/Mazel, 1990).

38. See "Closer Look Strips Glory from Vietnam War 'Hero,' " *San Diego Evening Tribune*, October 10, 1989, cited in Michael Yapko, *Suggestions of Abuse* (New York: Simon & Schuster, 1994), 3.

39. Harriet E. Lerner, "The Hysterical Personality: A 'Woman's Disease'"

in *Women and Mental Health*, ed. Elizabeth Howell and Marjorie Bayes (New York: Basic Books, 1987), 205, 196.

40. Freud, "Extracts from the Fliess Papers," *Standard Edition of the Complete Works of Sigmund Freud*, 24 vols., trans. James Strachey (London: Hogarth Press, 1953–1974), 1:228. Hereafter abbreviated as *SE*.

41. Wilhelm Reich, *Character-Analysis*, 3d ed., trans. Theodore P. Wolfe (New York: Farrar Straus Giroux, 1949), 189.

42. Carroll Smith-Rosenberg, *Disorderly Conduct: Visions of Gender in Victorian America* (New York: Knopf, 1985), 331.

43. "The Storming of St. Pat's," *New York Times*, December 12, 1989, A24.

44. Jane Ussher, *Women's Madness: Misogyny or Mental Illness?* (New York and London: Harvester/Wheatsheaf, 1991), 169.

45. Lucien Israel, *L'hystérique, le sexe, et le médecin* (Paris: Masson, 1983), 60.

6. Hysterical Narratives

1. Libby Purves, "I Think I Was a Good and Faithful Wife," *The Times* (London), February 4, 1994, 15.

2. Charles Richet, "Les démoniaques d'aujourd'hui et d'aurefois," *La revue des deux mondes* 37 (1880), 348.

3. Francisque Sarcey, "Le mot et la chose," (1863), 261, quoted in Jacqueline Carroy-Thirard, "Hystérie, théâtre, littérature au dix-neuvième siècle," *Psychanalyse à l'université* (March 1982): 299 (my translation).

4. Jann Matlock, *Scenes of Seduction: Prostitution, Hysteria, and Reading Difference in Nineteenth-Century France* (New York: Columbia University Press, 1994), 126–27.

5. Claire Kahane, "Hysteria, Feminism, and the Case of *The Bostonians*," in *Feminism and Psychoanalysis*, ed. Richard Feldstein and Judith Roof (Ithaca: Cornell University Press, 1989), 286–88.

6. Pioneering work on this topic has been done by professor Michele Birnbaum, especially "Racial Hysteria," a paper presented at the MLA panel on Hysteria and Narrative, December 1992.

7. Max Nordau, *Degeneration*, ed. George L. Mossé (Lincoln: University of Nebraska Press, 1993), 15.

8. Sigmund Freud, *Studies in Hysteria*, *SE* 2:160–61.

9. Sigmund Freud, *Dora: An Analysis of a Case of Hysteria* (New York: Collier, 1963), 7, 10.

10. Steven Marcus, "Freud and Dora: Story, History, Case History," in Bernheimer and Kahane, eds., *In Dora's Case*, 79.

11. Peter Brooks, *Body Work: Objects of Desire in Modern Narrative* (Cambridge: Harvard University Press), 235.

12. John Forrester, *The Seductions of Psychoanalysis* (Cambridge: Cambridge University Press, 1990), 8.

13. Susan Katz, "Speaking Out Against the 'Talking Cure,'" *Women's Studies* 13 (1987): 297–324.

14. Hélène Cixous, "The Laugh of the Medusa," *New French Feminisms*, ed.

Elaine Marks and Isabelle de Courtivron (Amherst: University of Massachusetts Press, 1980), 257.

15. Elaine Hedges and Shelley Fisher Fishkin, *Listening to Silences: New Essays in Feminist Criticism* (New York: Oxford University Press, 1994), 3. My discussion of Tillie Olsen's work on feminist critical theory is indebted to Hedges and Fishkin, especially their introduction to the book.

16. Patricia Yeager, *Honey-Mad Women: Emancipating Strategies in Women's Writing* (New York: Columbia University Press, 1988), 153–54.

17. Janis Stout, quoted in Hedges and Fishkin, *Listening to Silences*, 5.

18. Toril Moi, *Feminist Theory and Simone de Beauvoir* (London: Basil Blackwell, 1990), 92.

19. Evans, *Fits and Starts*, 282.

20. Sandra M. Gilbert and Susan Gubar, *The Madwoman in the Attic* (New Haven: Yale University Press, 1979), 98, 99.

21. Alice Walker, *In Search of Our Mother's Gardens* (New York: Harcourt Brace Jovanovich, 1983), 232–33.

22. Jean O. Love, *Virginia Woolf* (Berkeley: University of California Press, 1977), 195.

23. Louise DeSalvo, *Virginia Woolf: The Impact of Childhood Sexual Abuse on Her Work* (London: The Woman's Press, 1989), 1, 13, 14, 234.

24. Jan Marsh, *Christina Rossetti: A Literary Biography* (London: Jonathan Cape, 1994), 258, 259.

25. Barbara White, "Neglected Areas: Wharton's Short Stories and Incest, Part II" *Edith Wharton Review*, 8 (Fall 1991): 6,7.

26. Maureen Freely, "Blowing Hot and Hotter," *The Observer Review*, July 16, 1995, 12.

27. Julia Kristeva, in Marks and de Courtivron, eds., *New French Feminisms*, 166.

28. Juliet Mitchell, "Psychoanalysis: Child Development and Femininity," in *Women: The Longest Revolution* (London: Virago, 1984), 289–90.

29. Mary Jacobus, *Reading Woman* (New York: Columbia University Press, 1986), 201.

30. Jill L. Matus, "St. Teresa, Hysteria, and *Middlemarch*," in *Journal of the History of Sexuality*, 1 (1990): 216.

31. Brooks, *Body Work*, 231–32.

32. Eve Kosofsky Sedgwick, "Preface," *The Coherence of Gothic Conventions* (New York: Methuen, 1986), vi.

33. Jacobus, *Reading Woman*, 197.

34. Diane Price Herndl, "The Writing Cure," *NWSA Journal*, 1 (1988): 68.

35. Jacobus, *Reading Woman*, 229.

36. Barbara Johnson, "Is Female to Male as Ground Is to Figure?" *Feminism and Psychoanalysis*, ed. Richard Feldstein and Judith Roof, (Ithaca: Cornell University Press, 1989), 255, 258.

37. Gillian Brown, "The Empire of Agoraphobia," *Representations*, 20 (Fall 1987): 152*n*3.

38. Michelle A. Massé, *In the Name of Love: Women, Masochism, and the Gothic* (Ithaca: Cornell University Press, 1992), 16.

39. Herndl, "The Writing Cure," 74.

40. Lisa Gornick, "Developing a New Narrative: The Woman Therapist and the Male Patient," in *Psychoanalysis and Women: Contemporary Reappraisals*, ed. Judith L. Alpert (Hillsdale, N.J.: The Analytic Press, 1986), 257–85.

41. See Casey Miller and Kate Swift, *Words and Women* (New York: Anchor Books, 1977), 60–61.

42. Sandra Gilbert and Susan Gubar, "The Man on the Dump versus the United Dames of America; or, What Does Frank Lentricchia Want?" *Critical Inquiry*, 14 (1988): 386–406.

43. Jan Goldstein, "The Uses of Male Hysteria: Medical and Literary Discourse in Nineteenth-Century France," *Representations*, 34 (Spring 1991): 143.

44. See Katz, "Speaking Out Against the 'Talking Cure.'"

45. "Interview with Pat Barker," in Donna Perry, *Backtalk: Women Writers Speak Out* (New Brunswick, N.J.: Rutgers University Press, 1993), 43–62.

46. Martin Amis, *The Sunday Times* (London), September 24, 1995.

7. Hysteria and the Histrionic

1. Jules Falret, *Etudes cliniques sur les maladies mentales et nerveuse* (Paris: Librairie Ballière et Fils, 1890), 502.

2. Jacqueline Carroy-Thirard, "Hystérie, théâtre, littérature au dix-neuvième siècle," *Psychanalyse à l'université*, 7 (March 1982): 302.

3. Georgette Déga, quoted in Martha Noel Evans, *Fits and Starts* (Ithaca: Cornell University Press, 1991), 72.

4. See the fascinating article by Rae Beth Gordon, "Le Caf'con et l'hystérie," *Romanticisme*, 64 (1989): 53–66.

5. Hélène Zimmern, "Eleanora Duse," *Fortnightly Review* (1900): 983, quoted in John Stokes, "The Legend of Duse," in *Decadence and the 1890s*, ed. Ian Fletcher (London: Edward Arnold, 1979), 162; and Michael Robinson, "Acting Women: The Performing Self and the Late Nineteenth Century," *Comparative Criticism*, 14 (1992): 3–24.

6. Elin Diamond, "Realism and Hysteria: Toward a Feminist Mimesis," *Discourse*, 13 (Fall–Winter 1990–91): 63.

7. Harry Campbell, *Differences in the Nervous Organization of Man and Woman: Physiological and Pathological* (London, H.K. Lewis, 1891), 169.

8. See also Felicia McCarren, "The 'Symptomatic Act' Circa 1900: Hysteria, Hypnosis, Electricity, Dance," *Critical Inquiry*, 21 (Summer 1995): 748–74.

9. Sigmund Freud and Josef Breuer, "Fraulein Anna O.," *Studies on Hysteria* (New York: Avon, 1966), 76.

10. Kay H. Blacker and Joe P. Tupin, "Hysteria and Hysterical Structures: Development and Social Theories," in Mardi J. Horowitz, ed., *Hysterical Personality* (New York: Jason Aronson, 1977), 130.

11. Gunnar Brandell, *Freud: A Man of His Century*, trans. Ian White, (Hassock: Harvester Press, 1979), 35, 38. See Lis Muller, "The Analytical Theatre: Freud and Ibsen," *Scandinavian Psychoanalytic Review*, 13 (1990): 113.

12. Max Nordau, *Degeneration*, ed. George L. Mosse (Lincoln: University of Nebraska Press, 1993), 414.

13. Ibsen, 166.

14. Charles Spencer, *Daily Telegraph*, May 9, 1991.

15. John Peter, *Sunday Times*, June 30, 1991.

16. Fiona Shaw, Celebritea discussion, Royal National Theatre, London, August 20, 1993.

17. Fiona Shaw, "The Post-Feminist Myth," *the sphinx* (London: Sadler's Wells, 1991), 53.

18. See reviews of *Hedda Gabler*, by Michael Billington, *The Guardian*, September 5, 1991; Maureen Paton, *Daily Express*, September 5, 1991; Rhoda Koenig, *Punch*, September 11, 1991; Milton Shulman, *Evening Standard*, September 4, 1991, and Christopher Edwards, *Spectator*, September 7, 1991.

19. Kerry Powell, *Wilde and the Theatre of the 1890s* (Cambridge: Cambridge University Press, 1990), 79.

20. Mann, *Richard Strauss: A Critical Study of the Operas* (London: Cassell, 1964), 50–51.

21. Sander L. Gilman, *Disease and Representation: Images of Illness From Madness to AIDS* (Ithaca: Cornell University Press, 1988), 168–69.

22. See Janet Walker, *Couching Resistance: Women, Film, and Psychoanalytic Theory* (Minneapolis: University of Minnesota Press, 1993), 52.

23. Don Black and Christopher Hampton, *Sunset Boulevard* (London and Boston: Faber and Faber, 1993), 26.

24. See McCarren, "The 'Symptomatic Act,'" 772–73.

25. Dianne Hunter, "Representing Mad Contradictoriness in *Dr. Charcot's Hysteria Shows*," *Themes in Drama*, ed. James Redmond (Columbia University Press, 1993), 101.

26. Mady Schutzman, "Dr. Charcot's Hysteria Shows," in *Women & Performance* 5 (1990): 183–89.

27. Evans, *Fits and Starts*, 216, 217.

28. Judith Roof, "Marguerite Duras and the Question of a Feminist Theater," in Feldstein and Roof, *Feminism and Psychoanalysis* (Ithaca: Cornell University Press, 1989), 327.

29. Kim Morrissey, *Dora: A Case of Hysteria* (London: Nick Hern Books, 1994), 30.

30. See Elaine Showalter, " 'Mrs. Klein': The Mother, the Daughter, the Thief, and Their Critics," *Woman: A Cultural Review* I (Summer 1990), 144–48.

31. Paul Taylor, "It's the Way We Tell 'em," *The Independent*, April 6, 1994, 25.

32. Lizzie Francke, "Funny Girls," *The Guardian*, April 12, 1994, 17.

33. Hélène Cixous and Catherine Clément, *The Newly Born Woman* (Minneapolis: University of Minnesota Press, 1975), trans. Betsy Wing, 13.

34. See Paul Smith, "Action Movie Hysteria, or Eastwood Bound," *Differences*, 1 (1989): 103, 105.

35. Barbara Creed, "Phallic Panic: Male Hysteria and *Dead Ringers*," *Screen*, 31 (Summer 1991): 133.

36. Lynne Kirby, "Male Hysteria and Early Cinema," *Camera Obscura* 17 (1991), 124, 128.

37. Ed Sikov, *Laughing Hysterically: American Screen Comedy of the 1950s* (New York: Columbia University Press, 1994), 190–91.

8. Chronic Fatigue Syndrome

1. Olivia Fane, "He Said: You Can Walk. And She Could," *The Independent*, April 4, 1994, 18.

2. Liz Hunt, "Despair in a Doll's House," *The Independent*, May 17, 1994, 19.

3. J. Seligmann, P. Abranson, P. Shapiro, D. Gosnell, and M. Hager, "The Malaise of the Eighties," *Newsweek*, October 7, 1986, 105–6.

4. Anthony K. Komaroff, "Clinical Presentation and Evaluation of Fatigue in CFS," in *Chronic Fatigue Syndrome*, ed. Stephen E. Straus (New York: Marcel Dekker, 1994), 61.

5. Luisa Dillner, "Doctor at Large: Inject Some Fun to Beat Fatigue," *The Guardian*, May 19, 1995, 10.

6. Arthur Kleinman and Stephen Straus, "Introduction," *Chronic Fatigue Syndrome*, proceedings of CIBA conference, May 12–14, 1992 (London: Wiley, 1993), 3.

7. Karyn Feiden, *Hope and Help for Chronic Fatigue Syndrome* (New York: Simon and Schuster, 1990), 3.

8. Komaroff, "Clinical Presentation," 52.

9. Simon Wessely, in *Chronic Fatigue Syndrome* (London: Wiley, 1993), 338.

10. See also Hillary Johnson, "Journey Into Fear," *Rolling Stone*, July 16 and August 13, 1987.

11. "America's Next Epidemic," ad for *Osler's Web* in *New York Times Book Review*, March 31, 1996, 5.

12. Hillary Johnson, *Osler's Web* (New York: Crown, 1996), 6.

13. Feiden, *Hope and Help for Chronic Fatigue Syndrome*, 29.

14. Johnson, *Osler's Web*, 33.

15. Jon Kaplan, quoted in Johnson, *Osler's Web*, 51.

16. Simon Wessely, "New Wine in Old Bottles: Neurasthenia and 'ME,'" *Psychological Medicine*, 20 (1990): 35–53.

17. "Neurasthenia and Modern Life," *British Medical Journal*, 1909, cited in ibid., 44.

18. Wessely, "New Wine," 47.

19. Johnson, *Osler's Web*, 118.

20. Simon Wessely, "The History of Chronic Fatigue Syndrome," in Stephen E. Straus, ed., *Chronic Fatigue Syndrome* (New York: Marcel Dekker, 1994), 29.

21. Johnson, *Osler's Web*, 50, 65–66, 138.

22. Hillary Johnson, "Journey Into Fear," *Rolling Stone*, 16 July and 13 August 1987.

23. David S. Bell, *The Doctor's Guide to Chronic Fatigue Syndrome* (Boston: Addison-Wesley, 1995), 8–9.

24. Feiden, *Hope and Help*, 63–65.

25. *USA Today*, February 1993.

26. Neenyah Ostrom, *What Really Killed Gilda Radner? Frontline Reports on the Chronic Fatigue Syndrome* (New York: TNM, 1989).

27. Ryan Murphy, "Whatever Happened to Cher?" *McCall's*, May 1994, 108–111.

28. Betsy Kraus, *Library Journal*, June 15, 1992, 94.

29. Wessely, "History of Chronic Fatigue Syndrome," 24.

30. Wessely, "New Wine," 20.

31. Lawrence B. Altman, "Study Ties Chronic Fatigue Syndrome to Abnormality in the Control of Blood Pressure," *New York Times*, September 27, 1995, A16.

32. Bell, *The Doctor's Guide to Chronic Fatigue Syndrome*, 232.

33. Quoted in Johnson, *Osler's Web*, 146.

34. Deanne Pearson, "Unwillingly to School," *Times* (London), August 20, 1995, 23.

35. Johnson, *Osler's Web*, 612, 629.

36. Review of Timothy P. Kenny, *Living With Chronic Fatigue Syndrome: A Personal Story of the Struggle for Recovery*, *Publishers Weekly*, March 4, 1994, 69.

37. Gail MacLean and Simon Wessely, "Professional and Popular Views of Chronic Fatigue Syndrome," *British Medical Journal* 308 (March 19, 1994): 776–77.

38. Wessely, "The History of Chronic Fatigue Syndrome," 39.

39. See Komaroff, "Clinical Presentation."

40. Bell, *The Doctor's Guide*, 52–53.

41. Wessely, "New Wine," 39.

42. Edward Shorter, *From Paralysis to Fatigue* (New York: The Free Press, 1992), 317.

43. See Johnson, *Osler's Web*, 348, and ibid., 317, for examples.

44. Johnson, *Osler's Web*, 680.

45. Carol Midgley and Liz Jenkins, "BBC Defends Rantzen Over TV 'Shout-in' Claim," The *Times*, August 7, 1996, 5.

46. Victor Lewis-Smith, "A Paid-up Member of the ME Generation," *Evening Standard*, August 6, 1996, 27.

47. Lisa O'Carroll and Nick Pryer, "Trial by TV for the Doctor Who Dared to Disagree with Esther," *Evening Standard*, August 6, 1996, 3.

48. Cited in Johnson, *Osler's Web*, 260, 684–85.

49. Arthur Kleinman, in Straus, ed., *Chronic Fatigue Syndrome* (London: Wiley, 1993), 258, 329.

50. David Mechanic, in Straus, ed., *Chronic Fatigue Syndrome*, 327–28.

51. Wessely, "New Wine," 50.

52. Johnson, *Osler's Web*, 684.

53. Deanne Pearson, "Unwillingly to School," 23.

54. Johnson, *Osler's Web*, 680.

9. Gulf War Syndrome

1. David France, "The Families Who Are Dying for Our Country," *Redbook*, September 1994, 117.

2. Ibid., 116.

3. Melanie McFadyean, "Soldier On," *The Guardian Weekend*, May 27, 1995, 25 ff.

4. Gregory Jaynes, "Walking Wounded," *Esquire*, May 1994, 74.

5. France, "Families," 148.

6. Jaynes, "Walking Wounded," 71.

7. Edward Pilkington, "Gulf War Veterans Fear for their Families," *The Guardian*, June 12, 1995, 4.

8. Jaynes, "Walking Wounded," 71.

9. Jonathan Freedland, "Cover-up Alleged as US Denies Gulf War Syndrome Exists," *The Guardian*, August 3, 1995, 2.

10. France, "Families," 148.

11. Ibid., 116.

12. Quoted in Kenneth Miller, "The Tiny Victims of Desert Storm," *Life*, November 1995, 62.

13. Jaynes, "Walking Wounded," 73.

14. See Philip Shenon, "New Report Cited on Chemical Arms Used in Gulf War," *New York Times*, August 22, 1996, A1, B13.

15. France, "Families," 147.

16. Scott Allen, "Gulf Troops Received Experimental Drug," *Boston Sunday Globe*, July 3, 1994, 1, 16.

17. France, "Families," 116.

18. "Report Offers No One Cause for Gulf War Illness," *New York Times*, December 14, 1994.

19. Philip J. Hilts, "Study on Ailing Gulf War G.I.s Called a Failure," *New York Times*, January 5, 1995.

20. "Study of 19,000 Finds No 'Gulf War Syndrome,'" *New York Times*, April 4, 1996, B11.

21. David Fairhall, "Gulf War 'Fever' Rejected by MoD," *The Guardian*, June 8, 1995.

22. Michael Evans, "Gulf War Syndrome Inquiry Supported," *The Times*, July 28, 1995, 4.

23. Simon Wessely, "What Is This Mystery Illness Which We Call Gulf War Syndrome?" *The Times*, July 27, 1995.

24. Laura Flanders, "Bringing the War Home," *The Women's Review of Books*, 11 (July 1994): 10.

25. Laura Flanders, "A Lingering Sickness," *The Nation*, January 23, 1995, 96.

26. Ibid., 96.

27. Miller, "Tiny Victims," 46–62.

28. Jaynes, "Walking Wounded," 75.

29. France, "Families," 147–48.

30. Ibid., 147.

31. "Comprehensive Clinical Evaluation Program (CCEP) for Gulf War Veterans," Department of Defense, August 1995.

32. Wessely, "What Is This Mystery Illness?"

33. Scott Allen, "Gulf Troops," 1, 16.

34. Statement to Committee, September 29, 1992, *Illness of Persian Gulf Veterans*, serial no. 102–51, U.S. Government Printing Office, Washington, D.C., 1993, 84.

35. Flanders, "Bringing the War Home," 10.

36. Joseph P. Kennedy, Monday, September 21, 1992, in *Illness of Persian Gulf Veterans*, 30.

37. Paul Cotton, "Veterans Seeking Answers to Syndrome Suspect They Were Goats in Gulf War," *JAMA* 271 (1994), 1559, 1561.

38. Richard A. Kulka et al., *Trauma and the Vietnam War Generation* (New York: Brunner/Mazel, 1990), 232.

10. Recovered Memory

1. Judith Lewis Herman, *Trauma and Recovery* (New York: Basic Books, 1992), 28.

2. Bessel A. Van der Kolk and Onno Van der Hart, "The Intrusive Past: The Flexibility of Memory and the Engraving of Trauma," in *Trauma*, ed. Cathy Carruth (Baltimore: Johns Hopkins University Press, 1995), 176.

3. Herman, *Trauma and Recovery*, 122.

4. Ibid., 178, 188. The term *unstory* comes from Lawrence Langer, *Holocaust Testimonies: The Ruins of Memory* (New Haven: Yale University Press, 1991), 39.

5. Herman, *Trauma and Recovery*, 185–86.

6. Louise Armstrong, *Rocking the Cradle of Sexual Politics: What Happened When Women Said Incest* (London: The Woman's Press, 1996), 4, 210.

7. Katy Butler, "You Must Remember This," *The Guardian*, July 23, 1994.

8. Frederick Crews, *The Memory Wars: Freud's Legacy in Disrepute* (New York: New Yale Review Books, 1995), 159.

9. Richard Webster, *Why Freud Was Wrong* (New York: Basic Books, 1995), 511.

10. Armstrong, *Rocking the Cradle*, 207.

11. Claudette Wassil-Grimm, *Diagnosis for Disaster* (Woodstock, N.Y.: Overlook Press, 1995), 350.

12. See Elizabeth Loftus and Katherine Ketcham, *The Myth of Repressed Memory: False Memories and Allegations of Sexual Abuse* (New York: St. Martin's Press), 1994.

13. Michael Yapko, *Suggestions of Abuse: True and False Memories of Childhood Sexual Trauma* (New York: Simon & Schuster, 1994), 20.

14. Richard Ofshe and Ethan Watters, *Making Monsters: False Memories, Psychotherapy, and Sexual Hysteria* (New York: Scribner's, 1994), 305–12.

15. Ellen Bass and Laura Davis, *The Courage to Heal*, 2d ed. (New York: Harper Perennial, 1992), 107.

16. Ibid., 24.

17. Armstrong, *Rocking the Cradle*, 52n.; Diane Russell, *The Secret Trauma* (New York: Basic Books, 1986), 10.

18. Ofshe and Watters, *Making Monsters*, 48.

19. Lisa Watts, "The Career Price of Sexual Abuse," *Harvard Magazine* (October 1994): 18, 20.

20. Mike Lew, *Victims No Longer* (London: Cedar, 1993), 55, 57.

21. Ibid., 69, 152.

22. Bass and Davis, *The Courage to Heal*, 3d ed., 410.

23. Ibid., 532.

24. Rebecca Peppler Sinkler, "Picks, Pans, and Fragile Egos," *Civilization* (July/August 1995): 51.

25. Judith Herman, "Backtalk," *Mother Jones* (March/April 1993): 4.

26. Katy Butler, "Did Daddy Really Do It?" *Los Angeles Times Book Review*, February 5, 1995, 11.

27. Carol Tavris, "Beware the Incest-Survivor Machine," *New York Times Book Review*, January 3, 1993; see Ofshe and Watters, *Making Monsters*, 200.

11. Multiple Personality Syndrome

1. Ian Hacking, *Rewriting the Soul: Multiple Personality and the Sciences of Memory* (Princeton: Princeton University Press, 1995), 39.

2. Flora Rheta Schreiber, *Sybil* (New York: Warner, 1973), 5, and Mark Pendergrast, *Victims of Memory: Incest Accusations and Shattered Lives* (Hinesburg, Vt.: Upper Access, 1995), 155.

3. See Hacking, *Rewriting the Soul*, 51–52.

4. Richard Kluft, "Treatment of Multiple Personality Disorder: A Study of Thirty-Three Cases," *Psychiatric Clinics of North America*, 7 (1984): 69–88.

5. G. B. Greaves, "President's Letter," *Newsletter of the International Society for the Study of Multiple Personality & Dissociation*, 5 (1987): 1; quoted in Hacking, *Rewriting the Soul*, 52.

6. C. A. Ross, "Epidemiology of Multiple Personality Disorder and Dissociation," *Psychiatric Clinics of North America*, 14 (1991): 503–18

7. Colin Ross, quoted in Richard Ofshe and Ethan Watters, *Making Monsters: False Memories, Psychotherapy, and Sexual Hysteria*, 206.

8. Ray Aldridge-Morris, *Multiple Personality: An Exercise in Delusion* (London: Lawrence Erlbaum, 1989), and Harold Merskey, "The Manufacture of Personalities: The Production of Multiple Personality Disorder," *British Journal of Psychiatry*, 160 (1992): 337.